Doctor Silvers'

Extraordinary
Remedies and Prescriptions
for Health and Longevity

Doctor Silvers'

PRENTICE-HALL, INC.

Englewood Cliffs, N.J.

Extraordinary
Remedies and Prescriptions
for Health and Longevity

Lewis J. Silvers, M.D.

PRINTED IN THE UNITED STATES OF AMERICA

21866—B & P

IN MEMORY OF

Miriam and Lori

How Doc Silvers
Will Help You to Help Yourself
to Healthy, Zestful Living

The trouble with life is that it often takes a lifetime to learn how to live. The adult frequently sighs and says, "If I only knew years ago what I know now." This particularly applies to the state of one's health. Modern man, civilized and intelligent though he may be, is vastly ignorant about the wonders of his own body. He knows little or nothing of the natural forces which, despite the ill treatment he gives it, keep him alive and in reasonably good health. I am constantly amazed that man, with his lack of knowledge of the simplest principles of Nature, hasn't disappeared from the face of the earth eons ago.

Will man survive? I have often had my doubts, but I still believe that he will. However, he can only do so by learning and obeying the laws of Nature. And the sooner he does so, the better chance he has of survival. Today millions suffer needlessly because they do not know the fundamental rules of health. And the tragedy of it is they are so simple that even primitive man understood them. He knew that natural forces: water, light, heat and air, could relieve his aches and pains, and frequently cure many of his numerous ills.

Why then are we, his descendants, millions of years later, so ignorant of these natural laws? We rely upon pills and potions, and we expect psychiatrists to cure us of our deep-seated neuroses with the wave of a magic wand. But we do little or nothing for ourselves!

7

Does that make sense? Of course not. We want medicine to work wonders, and it does. However, good health basically depends on how you care for and treat your own body through the years. Your family physician does everything possible to keep you well, yet the responsibility for observing the principles of health rests upon your own shoulders. And that is precisely where it belongs!

It has taken nearly half a century of preparation before I could write this book. During those many fruitful years, I became more and more convinced, as Robert Burns put it, of "man's inhumanity to man," particularly with regard to his own health and well-being. Man, despite his cruelties, is often a Good Samaritan to the weary wayfarer, but not to himself. He goes through life thoughtlessly, as if it were a trip around Disneyland. He treats his body, which he cannot replace, as if it were a cloak he could remove at will. It has to fight valiantly to stave off the follies he forces upon it. Day after day, Nature struggles to keep this marvelous mechanism from being destroyed through sheer neglect.

How much attention and care do you give to the physical structure which houses your heart and soul? Do you look at it with admiration and respect, as you should? Do you keep it in as good repair as your home and your car? A house and a car need more than a new paint job now and then; and your body deserves far more.

The purpose of therapeutics is to heal and cure. But the ultimate aim of medicine is to raise the standards of health of all humanity. One important way to reach this goal is to inform people how to keep themselves well. And that is the prime purpose of this book. In these pages, I propose to demonstrate in lay language just exactly what you can do to further your good health by preventions, remedies, and other means, all of which can be practised at home in the natural surroundings of everyday living, easily, simply, and at little or no cost.

This book is the culmination of over forty years of medical practice. During that protracted period, I have prescribed hundreds of preventions and remedies for use in the home to thousands of patients. Now it is my earnest desire to pass these treatments on to many more thousands beyond my immediate sphere of influence so they also may benefit by them. They are all simple, and they are all safe, having been tested in the crucible of experience. They are yours to "use as directed," as the label on prescriptions commonly states. The reports from many of my patients over the years prove that they have benefited, and they will work for you, as well. In following them, you will feel healthier, stronger, younger; you will prevent the inception of many minor, and even major, illnesses; you will remedy numerous maladies; you will look better, feel better, and retard the advancing years; you will be happier, have more fun, and appreciably extend the useful and enjoyable years of life to a ripe old age. All you need do to gain these appreciable rewards is to observe the simply understandable principles of good health.

Doc Silvers says: "The best way to maintain healthfulness of body and mind—as Hippocrates, the father of medicine, advised nearly two thousand years ago—is to follow the laws of Nature."

Contents

Uncommon Remedies for Common Ailments   17

1. Why This Book Will Be so Easy to Use   25
   sister kenny's "miracle cure", 25 · why the simple way is usually the best way, 28 ·

2. How to Use Heat and Cold to Cure Your Ills   31
   how increased circulation can increase your health, 32 · applying compresses, 33 · using salt solutions in hot compresses, 33 · how to use compresses most effectively, 34 ·

3. Using Light and Massage for Greater Comfort and Ease   37
   advantages of light therapy, 37 · understanding how light therapy works, 38 · how light affects your skin, 38 · how sunbathing can help and hurt you, 39 · avoid sunburn of the eyes, 40 · using infrared light at home, 42 · how to use home massage effectively, 42 · muscle cramp, 43 ·

4. Nude Bathing for Good Health and Healthy Skin   49
   nudity isn't shameful, 51 · the benefits of artificial sunlight, 53 · how to select and use a sunlamp properly, 54 · give your skin the nutrition it needs, 54 ·

5. Bathing Remedies to Get Lasting Results   57

gain those big benefits of water therapy, 57 · how to use cold-water therapy, 58 · how to use hot-water therapy, 59 · why you should water the tree of life, 61 · effective salt water bathing at home, 62 · how ocean bathing can pay big dividends, 63 · using climato-therapy for better health, 64 · are you "discomfort-able?", 65 · know how to play it safe, 66 ·

6. How to Use the Sun as a Master Medicine   69

how to get instant relief from insect bites, 70 · a dozen ways to beat the heat, 71 · air bathing in the nude, 71 · how climate influences your health, 73 · what to do about the weather, 75 ·

7. Activities and Exercises as Rejuvenators, Restoratives, and Invigorators   77

don't force yourself, 77 · the right way to breathe, 78 · belly breathing, 78 · what belly breathing does for you, 79 · you can swim your way to better health, 80 · exercise after your shower, 81 · how to make a prog-ress report, 86 · enjoy yourself more by being fit, 88 ·

8. Putting More Spice in Your Life by Putting More Variety in Your Diet   91

natural foods to make you feel better, 92 · how to avoid insecticides, 93 · why the staff of life can be life-less, 93 · raw vs. cooked foods as a health measure, 94 · know when to eat, 96 · learn to use natural laxatives, 98 · don't be a worry wart, 100 · don't be a slave to laxatives, 100 ·

9. How to Lose Weight without Losing Vigor   103

reduce gradually, 103 · reduce one pound a week, 103 · know your desirable weight, 104 · how to deter-mine your daily calorie allowance, 105 · how to reduce without starving, 107 · recognize these protein protectors, 108 · use this prudent diet, 109 · vary your menus, 110 · why your biggest enemy is your sweet tooth, 113 · avoid bread and butter and lose 28 pounds, 113 · summarizing your pound-a-week program, 113 · how advances in food processing can keep you thinner, 114 · dietary of the future, 118 ·

10. How to Relax without Drugs   119

learn to relax, 120 · get up with the birds, 119 · hot vs. cold drinks, 122 · quick cure for indigestion, 123 · an easy way to avoid nausea, 124 · how to relieve peptic indigestion, 124 · a three-way cocktail, 125 ·

11. How to Get to Sleep Faster and Rest Easier   129

you don't need sleep, 130 · should you take sleeping pills, 130 · how to tell a habit from an addiction, 132 · how to get easier sleep and more rest, 134 · hot drinks make sleepy people, 135 · try a tranquilizing tub, 135 · how to unlax your muscles, 136 ·

12. Treating Common Skin Disorders without Costly Drugs and Cosmetics   139

why cosmetics aren't always necessary, 140 · how to avoid scaly skin, 142 · treatment for poison ivy, 143 · how to treat burns quickly and effectively, 145 · treating pimples and boils, 151 · how to treat and protect minor skin injuries, 153 · how your skin reflects your general health, 154 ·

13. How to Avoid Nose Ailments   155

how your nose governs other body functions, 156 · treatment of sinus infection and headache, 157 · what you need to know about colds, 160 ·

14. How to Prevent and Treat Sore Throats   167

how to make your own cough medicine, 167 ·

15. Techniques for Safeguarding Your Sight   177

    how nature protects your eyes, 177 · don't waste beef steak on shiners, 178 ·

16. Easy Ways to Protect Your Hearing   187

    treatments for motion sickness and migraine, 189 ·

17. How to Feel Young, Stay Young, and Live Longer   195

    don't argue unnecessarily, 199 · how to achieve harmonious sexual intimacy in marriage, 200 · helping women over their difficult days, 201 ·

Index   207

Doctor Silvers'

Extraordinary
Remedies and Prescriptions
for Health and Longevity

UNCOMMON REMEDIES AND PREVENTIONS FOR COMMON AILMENTS

A quick reference guide to the use of this book.

AILMENT	RX	REFERENCE READING
Abscess	1 tbsp Epsom Salt, 1 tsp Bicarbonate of Soda, 1 pt hot water. Dip compress in solution, wring out, and apply until cool. Dip compress in solution again and reapply until swelling subsides and pain is relieved. After a few days of this treatment, abscess should open of itself, thus avoiding surgery.	Chapter 2
Acne	Expose affected area to sun 15 minutes a day, or use sunlamp in accordance with instructions.	Chapter 4
Atherosclerosis	To prevent atherosclerosis, take 1 or 2 tbsp cod liver oil, corn, cottonseed, safflower, or peanut oil daily, and 1 tbsp each lecithin (soya bean powder) and brewer's yeast daily.	Chapter 8 & Chapter 9

17

AILMENT	RX	REFERENCE READING
Athlete's foot	Borated talcum or Undecylenic Acid powder. Dry feet and put between toes after bathing.	Chapter 12
Baldness	Cut down starch, fat, and sugar in diet. Shampoo with Aveeno Soap Cake. Don't wear hats, especially tight ones.	Chapter 12
Black Eye	Cleanse eye with boric acid solution, then place cold compresses of boric acid solution over eye for period of one hour. Repeat applications one hour on, one hour off, until redness and pain subside.	Chapter 15
Boils	Apply swabbings of iodine for 1 full minute. Repeat morning and night.	Chapter 12
Burns	Salt solution of 1 tsp common salt and 1 pt cold water. Apply to area with saturated sterile gauze.	Chapter 12
Canker sores	Have druggist make up a solution of: Resublimed Iodine crystals 0.1, Potassium Iodine 3.0, Sol. Guaiicol 5.0, Essence Peppermint 1.0, honey or glycerine q.s. 100.0. Apply to sores with cotton applicator.	Chapter 14
Circulation	Poor circulation may be stimulated by having someone apply petrissage massage to the muscles of arms and legs, always working from the lower part up toward	

heart. Pick up flesh between thumb and finger, keeping thumb rigid, and roll flesh against it with fingers. Then keep fingers rigid, and roll flesh against them with thumb. Alternate these movements a half-dozen times. Repeat until entire muscle has been massaged.

Chapter 3

Colds

1 2-grain quinine pill every 4 hours, followed by hot drink of juice ½ lemon, 2 tbsp honey, 200 mg. Vitamin C, in glass of boiled water.

Chapter 13

Constipation

1 tbsp malt soup extract up to 3 times daily, mixed with milk, soup, or fruit juice.

Chapter 8

Coughs

Have druggist make up a solution of Resublimed Iodine Crystals 0.1, Potassium Iodide 3.0, Sol. Guaiicol 5.0, Essence Peppermint 1.0, honey q.s. 100.0. Swab on mucus membranes of mouth and throat.

Chapter 14

Dry scalp

Part hair and apply small amount lanolin cream to scalp, rubbing in with fingertips. Use daily.

Chapter 12

Dry skin

1 capsule 25,000 units Vitamin A after breakfast each morning.

Chapter 12

Dust in eyes

Wash out with eyecup of clean salt water: 1 tsp salt to 1 pt boiled, cold water. Follow with boric acid solution.

Chapter 15

AILMENT	RX	REFERENCE READING
Earache	2 or 3 drops pure glycerine, slightly warmed. Apply with dropper.	Chapter 16
Ear infection	To avoid ear infection, blow nose gently, with head forward, mouth open, and nostrils unobstructed.	Chapter 13
Ear wax	½ dropper peroxide in each ear at bedtime. Plug ears with cotton overnight.	Chapter 16
Eye strain	Blink eyes rapidly several times for natural lubrication. Do not use eyewash for this condition.	Chapter 15
Halitosis	1 tsp Aromatized Sodium Perborate in ½ glass warm water. Use as rinse morning and evening.	Chapter 14
Hay fever	½ percent of Neosynephrine in 1 oz dropper bottle, two drops in each nostril every four hours for temporary relief.	Chapter 13
Headache	Use effleurage massage for simple headache. Have someone stroke the forehead lightly with fingertips of one hand. Make a long stroke across forehead, then glide fingers back over skin to starting point. Continue until whole forehead has been covered, when headache will be relieved.	Chapter 3

Hives	Ask your pharmacist for an anti-histaminic, no prescription required. Take as directed and rash will disappear in ten days or less.	Chapter 12
Indigestion	Drink 3 drops Essence Peppermint mixed in ½ glass hot water.	Chapter 10
Inflammation	1 tbsp epsom salt, 1 tsp Bicarbonate of Soda, 1 pt ice-cold water. Saturate small cloth in solution, wring out, and apply to inflamed area for ½ hour. Soak cloth again and reapply until pain and swelling are reduced.	Chapter 2
Insect bites	Immediately apply a cotton swab saturated in Aromatic Spirits of Ammonia to the painful spot, which will relieve the pain at once.	Chapter 6
Insecticides on food	1 oz (2 tbsp) hydrochloric acid in 1 qt cold water. Immerse any fruit and vegetables to be eaten raw in solution for 30 minutes. Rinse.	Chapter 8
Insomnia	1 tbsp honey and 1 tsp lemon juice in glass hot boiled water at bedtime.	Chapter 11
Itching skin	Adults: 3 to 4 tbsp Aveeno Oilated in tub of warm water (103°F).	Chapter 12
Laryngitis	1 tbsp lemon juice, 2 tbsp honey (or glycerin,) 2 tablets aspirin, 8 oz boiled hot water, mixed until aspirins dissolve. When comfort-	

AILMENT	RX	REFERENCE READING
	ably warm, gargle and expectorate, then gargle and swallow.	Chapter 14
Migraine	1 50 mg niacin vitamin tablet. Repeat in 10 minutes, if necessary.	Chapter 16
Muscle cramp	Stretch limb with quick jerk, which may knock out cramp. If not, rub muscle strongly for minute or two. Should pain persist, apply moist or dry heat.	Chapter 3
Nervous tension	Hot drink ½ hour before meal: tea, coffee, prune juice, bouillon.	Chapter 10
Pain in muscles or joints	Fill small cloth bag, about 6 inches square, with flaxseed, and sew up opening. Steep in very hot water for a few minutes. Allow to cool enough not to burn skin, and apply to painful area. Keep on one hour, off one hour, and continue until pain is relieved.	Chapter 5
Peptic indigestion	2 tsp vinegar, 1 tbsp honey. Mix in glass of hot water and drink slowly.	Chapter 10
Pimples	Apply iodine locally and repeatedly during 1st 24 hours.	Chapter 12
Pink eye	Bathe eye with boric acid solution. Drop two drops 10 percent Argyrol solution in eye.	Chapter 15

Poison Ivy	2 fluids oz *rhus toxicodendrum*, taken in milk, one drop a day, gradually working up to twenty drops, until entire amount is used. Taken in spring, provides immunity all summer.	Chapter 12
Poor appetite	Increase intake of vitamin C from citrus fruits, other fruits and vegetables.	Chapter 8
Scaly elbows	Avoid soap when washing and apply cold cream daily.	Chapter 12
Seasickness	Stroke downward from back of ears with fingers of hands, to upper part of neck, and along sides of each jaw. Also effective in nausea from other methods of travel.	Chapter 10
Sinus infection	1 tbsp epsom salt, 1 tsp bicarbonate of soda, 1 pt ice-cold water. Dip cloth in solution, wring out excess, and apply. Change to hot compresses of same solution after 48 hours, applying for 15 minutes, twice daily.	Chapter 13
Skin injuries (minor)	Cleanse with peroxide and allow to air dry. Apply Phenolated Calamine solution and let dry. Keep free of covering.	Chapter 12
Skin rash	Expose affected area to the sun for 15 minutes a day, or use sunlamp as directed.	Chapter 4
Smoker's drip	1 tsp salt in 1 pt warm water, used as douche for post-nasal drip in nasal cavity	Chapter 13

AILMENT	RX	REFERENCE READING
Sore throat	1 tbsp lemon juice, 2 tbsp honey (glycerin for diabetics), 1 tablet aspirin, 8 oz boiled hot water, mixed until aspirin dissolves. When tepid, gargle and expectorate, then gargle and swallow.	Chapter 14
Stye	Apply penicillin or neomycin ophthalmic ointment.	Chapter 15
Trench mouth	Dissolve tsp of Perborate of Soda in glass of boiled water. When cool, use as mouth wash and gargle. Apply 2% Gentian Violet to gums with cotton applicator. Allow to dry, then chew Sulphathiazole Gum.	Chapter 14

Why This Book Will
Be so Easy to Use

1 Ever since time immemorial, our ancestors have used physical means to improve health and prolong life. They employed Nature's beneficences to great advantage. Today, with modern knowledge, better understanding, and specific application, we can use these means even more favorably. And what is most important is that they can be applied right in your own home.

Let us first understand what physical medicine is. Later we shall learn exactly what it can do for you. It is that branch of medicine which embraces the employment of the physical properties of certain elements for physical and occupational therapy in the diagnosis and treatment of disease.

These elements are: *Heat, Cold, Water, Light, Electricity, Exercise, Massage, Mechanical devices.*

The wonderful thing about physical medicine is that it is all so basically simple. Like a straight line, it is the shortest distance between two points: ailment and remedy. Physical medicine is direct treatment; there's no beating about the bush. When you have an affliction, you counteract it by applying a physical means, the effect of which is known. What could be simpler than that?

sister kenny's "miracle cure"

Here is a graphic illustration, which is well known throughout the medical world. You may remember, or have heard of, the wonderful work done by a registered nurse, Elizabeth Kenny—fondly known by her British title, "Sister Kenny"—in the early treatment of infantile paralysis (now called poliomyelitis or "polio" for short) some thirty years ago. This dread crippler had run rampant in epidemics all over the earth, paralyzing and destroying hundreds of thousands, especially children. At that time, there was no known preventive or cure, and medical savants were stumped on how to stop the ravages of this deadly, communicable disease.

Sister Kenny was working as a nurse in the back country districts of Queensland, Australia, when she encountered this killer. Devoted to her duty, she tried everything in the hope of affording relief to her young, suffering patients. Eventually, from all the varied methods then in vogue for the treatment of the excruciating pains in the involved muscles, she observed that hot moist compresses worked best. And finally she devised the simple method of avoiding the complication of muscle contraction by just applying hot wet blankets to the affected parts.

In 1933, Sister Kenny set up a clinic for the express purpose of treating polio in this way. Two years later, a royal commission of inquiry reported unfavorably on her method. However, in 1939, it was accepted for use in Australian hospitals. After that official recognition, the Sister Kenny technique remained the best type of treatment for spastic muscles throughout the years.

Later, she came to America, and supervised her hot wet blanket technique at a hospital in Minneapolis. To keep the blanket as hot as tolerable to the patient, a pail filled with water at a temperature too hot for comfortable handling was provided with an automatic wringer. The steaming hot blanket was wrung out and cooled by air exposure to maximum skin tolerance, and then wrapped around the affected parts. The resulting increase in blood flow carried off the products of inflammation, relaxed the muscles, and pain was soon relieved.

This back-breaking nursing care, requiring profound devotion to the patient, is now no longer required. The prevention of poliomyelitis with the Salk and Sabin vaccines will soon make this disease as uncommon as smallpox and diphtheria already are.

Doc Silvers says: "Physical therapy, since it uses natural methods and is simple in its technique, is well adapted for home treatment by the layman."

It is not well known, but a number of advances in medicine were made by laymen. I had occasion to mention this when, as president of the New York Society for Physical Medicine, I had the pleasure of introducing Sister Kenny at one of our monthly meetings. Frankly, I was in a quandary. At the time, these doctors had been trying a wide variety of drugs, including curare (which you may remember is used by South American natives to poison their arrows) in the attempt to lessen the spasms of muscles injured by polio. And here was a simple homespun woman, who was prepared to tell us doctors of something new in the treatment of such a puzzling disease as infantile paralysis. Remember, this was before the immunizing vaccines were developed.

How was I to introduce this country nurse to the erudite medicos? Luckily, the day before the meeting, my daughter Myra had read the life story of Sister Kenny in the *Reader's Digest*. "Why Dad," she exclaimed when she finished, "this reads exactly like the story about Florence Nightingale!" And that gave me the clue to my introduction.

The following day, I began by reminding my confreres of the many discoveries made in the field of medicine by lay persons. The ordinary folk of Persia used vaccination long before Dr. Jenner of England noted the cowpox on the hands of a dairymaid. In Elizabethan England, the use of foxglove for edema or dropsy was practiced by a so-called Shropshire witch. She gathered herbs by the light of the full moon and, making a concoction of them, successfully treated Queen Elizabeth. Only much later was it learned that the effective herb of all the plants she picked was foxglove, or digitalis, which is effectively used to this day in the treatment of heart failure and its accompanying dropsy. The blood pressure apparatus was first used by an English minister, who measured the pressure in the arteries of the neck of horses. The laryngoscope, which permits us to see the working of the larynx while phonating (speaking) was invented by a Spanish teacher of the voice. Milk sickness, a scourge in pioneering days, exterminating horses and cattle, was traced by the farmers themselves to snakeroot. The first to remove stone from the bladder was a Jesuit priest.

And now, I concluded, we had Sister Kenny, who devoted like Florence Nightingale to ministering to the sick and dying, had discovered how to apply physical medicine in treating the victims of infantile paralysis. After that brief exposition, Sister Kenny, a tall Amazon of a woman, required no further help from me. In a clear, strong voice, she explained her therapy in simple terms, while the gathering of doctors listened silently in appreciation and wonder.

These doctors were so immersed in the vast complexities which are the very nature of the medical profession that they hadn't thought of so elementary a treatment as wrapping a pain-wracked polio patient in hot wet blankets.

why the simple way is usually the best way

That's the way it is with physical medicine. You will find that all of the many preventions and remedies given in this book have a plain, unadulterated, homey aspect about them. Nevertheless, they are invariably based on sound medical therapeutics, which I will briefly explain as we go along, for I believe an intelligent person not only wants to know what to do, but why. All of the treatments are worked out directly from cause to effect, like that straight line I mentioned a while ago. There are many examples throughout this book, but here is just one for a starter:

Heat brought to the body will dilate the vessels and increase the flow of blood through the part to which it is applied.

I emphasize this fundamental point for it is a universal principle in physical therapeutics. Each element used: cold, water, light, electricity, exercise, massage, and heat, has a characteristic influence upon the body which can be prognosticated and controlled. In physical medicine you know what you are doing because you are dealing with Nature. If it were not for this basically important factor, home therapy of any kind at all would be an impossibility.

But since it *does* exist, there are many preventions and remedies which can be utilized by everyone in the home.

Getting back to our example of using heat to dilate blood vessels, it is of tremendous significance because of the therapeutic value of the natural benefits that invariably result from its application. We shall learn about them in the following chapter, where we detail the application of home treatments for a wide variety of ailments to which the human constitution is prone. Some of the techniques are old, some are new, and others have been developed in my own medical practice. Many of them, surprisingly enough, are not well known. For a single illustration from many, there is a simple specific which will stop the development of a migraine headache. And yet, outside of my own patients, I have never met any sufferer from these miserable attacks who knew about it. It is because of this general lack of knowledge of elementary physical therapeutics that I have long wanted to write this book, and to that end have collected over the years the variety of home treatments which it contains.

How to Use Heat & Cold
to Cure Your Ills

2 The application of heat dilates the vessels, thus increasing the flow of blood. Once you know that invariable physical reaction, you don't have to be a doctor to figure out that if heat expands, cold must contract. And you'd be absolutely right. Cold has the opposite effect of heat. Cold applications cause the contraction of blood vessels, thus slowing up the flow of blood in both time and volume. When you understand these two simple principles which underlie the response of the body tissues to heat and cold, you will have no difficulty in choosing the correct treatment for any given ailment.

In these and the other aptitudes of Nature—water, light, electricity, exercise, and massage—we are provided with the simple means of restoring health and prolonging life, which are of immense significance to our entire well being, physical and mental.

In the use of heat and cold—which are opposite poles of the same phenomenon: temperature—it has been found that each of the various types of application has certain definite effects, as follow:

Dry heat—superficial and local
Moist heat—penetrating and soothing
Dry cold—superficial and pain-relieving
Moist cold—penetrating and benumbing the tissue

Cold is ideal in acute inflammations, especially shortly after an injury, where the tissues are red, hot, and swollen. Moist cold compresses are best applied while at rest, leaving them in contact with the swollen tissue for 12 to 24 hours at a stretch.

Moist Cold Compress
1 tablespoon epsom salt
1 teaspoon bicarbonate of soda
1 pint of ice-cold water

Saturate a small towel or wash cloth in this solution, wring out the excess water, and apply to inflamed area for half an hour. Then soak again and reapply until pain and swelling are controlled.

how increased circulation can improve your health

Heat, as we have learned, increases the flow and volume of blood, which then passes through an affected organ. By stepping up the circulation in this way, we hasten the removal of products of inflammation much faster. Keep in mind that inflammation is the means by which your bodily tissues fight off invasion by foreign substances. It is, therefore, not a sign of worsening disease, but rather a sign of the struggle for recovery—the swelling, redness, and pain being indications of the fight which is progressing. The white cells (leukocytes), which are the scavenger cells of the blood system, are mobilized to engulf and devour the invaders. The final outcome of the conflict depends upon the ability of the protecting cells of the body to overcome the enemy organisms. The process of walling off the intruders begins at once. Absorption of the end-products of the battle causes a rise in temperature. This increase in fever is Nature's further mechanism for stimulating the body's reaction, providing a greater outpouring of the white cells. The immunity to disease is determined by this response. If the body can overcome the invader early enough to prevent much damage, the infection may be aborted, that is, stopped and rendered ineffectual. If, however, the battle progresses to pus formation, then medical aid is required to open the abscess and release its contents.

applying compresses

You can help Mother Nature appreciably in this dramatic struggle between health and disease. By the use of hot compresses, Nature will be aided in opening the abscess bluntly, thus avoiding the necessity of surgical incision. The medium used for this purpose is a hypertonic salt solution, which helps overcome inflammation in muscles and joints. A solution is said to be hypertonic when it contains mineral salts that make it denser than plain water. Hot water which is rich in minerals acts just like a hypertonic salt solution, and all of the noted spas throughout the world make use of this natural phenomenon.

using salt solutions in hot compresses

By the important physical process known as osmosis (the passing of a fluid through a membrane in the direction of more concentrated fluid), the less concentrated liquid in the tissues flows toward the externally applied denser mineral (hypertonic) solution via the semipermeable membranes of the tissue cells. Swelling and inflammation are thus reduced in the affected parts, and pain is relieved when the nerve endings are no longer impinged upon by the pressure of the increased products of inflammation. Soreness disappears with the decreased swelling, and the patient is relieved. This you can do right in your own home with the use of such common salts as epsom, sodium chloride (table salt), Glauber's salt, or plain bicarbonate of soda. The principle involved, remember, is that you are using a solution denser than the body tissues. The fluid which bathes all the bodily cells is normally 0.9% salt solution in concentration. This is called physiologic (natural) salt solution, which is obtained in similar strength by dissolving one level teaspoonful of salt in one pint of water. Therefore, to obtain a salt solution that is hypertonic, we must either increase the amount of salt used, or diminish the quantity of water. For practical purposes, and to avoid irritating a very sensitive skin, a combination of salts is used which is not only hypertonic, but also soothing to the skin.

Hot Hypertonic Salt Solution
(non-irritating)
1 tablespoon epsom salt
1 teaspoon bicarbonate of soda
1 pint hot water
Add ingredients to water and stir until dissolved.

The proportions given provide the most effective solution. Dip compress, wring out excess, and apply to the inflamed area, be it a joint, muscle or gland. When compress cools, dip and reapply. Continue this technique until swelling subsides and pain is relieved. I advise my patients to apply the hot compresses for at least 20 minutes, and repeat every four hours according to necessity. In sinus cases, the application of the hot hypertonic salt solution relieves the headache in short order; the ideal time is just before going to bed, assuring a restful and refreshing night's sleep.

You will gradually appreciate the efficacy of moist heat and hypertonic salt solution as your experience with this simple technique grows. Patience is essential when dealing with any inflammatory condition. The natural process of recovery is timed by the physical and chemical reactions taking place in the damaged tissues and, once recovery has started, you cannot hurry it. The process of repair will require the time needed for the scavenger cells to carry off the debris, and for the new tissues to replace the old and damaged cells.

how to use compresses most effectively

Cold compresses of hypertonic salt solution are used for the relief of any bruise or injury which causes swelling and pain. Use cold water from the tap and add ice cubes, if available. Apply compresses directly after injury, and continue for a period of days, if necessary. Remember that the applications should be intermittent, one hour on and a half-hour off, thus avoiding excessive contraction of the blood vessels. Doctors advantageously reduce the swelling and alleviate the pain in bone fractures by having this regimen followed for a day or so prior to immobilization with a cast.

In addition to the use of compresses, there are now many enzymes on the market which, because they speed up specific reactions, have a most salutary effect on the reduction of swelling and concomitant pain. Some are vegetable derivatives, others are organic or glandular in nature, and they are taken orally. The use of enzymes while applying the compresses hastens the process of repair and recovery. Ask your doctor about them, and he will prescribe an enzyme when needed.

Doc Silvers says: "Heat expands—cold contracts. Remember that, and you will always know how to take care of various bumps, bruises, and other common injuries."

Using Light and Massage
for Greater Comfort and Ease

3 We have seen that applications of heat or cold are very effective in the alleviation of a wide variety of ailments and injuries. In the previous chapter, we discussed the uses of moist heat in the form of compresses dipped in a hypertonic salt solution. Now we will extend our knowledge of the benefits of heat by turning to light therapy, which accomplishes the same purpose as wet heat, though in a different way.

advantages of light therapy

Light therapy has several advantages over moist heat. In the latter we have to heat water and make a solution; the compresses have to be dipped into the solution when they cool off; and as the solution cools, it has to be reheated. The application of light therapy, on the other hand, is much simpler. We either expose ourselves to sunlight, or we simply turn on an electric bulb. And since the heat remains constant, there is no need to reheat the source, as is required when using compresses. The intensity of sunlight, for the short period required, stays much the same; and with light bulbs, there is no variation at all. Therefore, light therapy is often preferable, though the nature of the injury must be taken into consideration. For example, you would never use light for treating a local condition in any area on or near the face because, even though you wear dark glasses, there is always the possibility of permanent injury to the eyes.

understanding how light therapy works

The biophysics of light therapy teaches us much about the way in which ultraviolet and infrared rays affect the bodily functions. When you are exposed to the sun's rays, you may be gradually tanned by carefully avoiding an overdose of sunshine at any single exposure. (Later we shall discuss sunbathing at length.) The skin becomes red because the blood vessels are dilated—heat expands them, remember? The exposure of the skin to the ultraviolet rays releases certain proteins into the blood stream. Among them is one known as histamine. The protein has the special property of causing the skin vessels to dilate. The normal presence of ergosterol in the skin is thus changed into viosterol or vitamin D. We now know that small amounts of this vitamin are essential daily for the normal function of the organs and bones of the body.

Regardless of the wave length of any form of radiation, a biologic effect can be observed only if its energy is transformed into heat. Ultraviolet radiation acts on cells in the same manner as radium or Roentgen rays. Applied in large doses, it retards growth and destroys any living substance. It is, however, much less penetrating, and so cannot do as much damage to living tissue. The use of light for sterilization is based on its destructive power. A short exposure to ultraviolet light will kill nearly all bacteria. Dwarfed vegetation in mountain climates is thus explained by the effect of increased exposure to ultraviolet, and not to lower temperatures and stronger prevailing winds, as was formerly believed.

how light affects your skin

The universal measurement of light is in Angstrom Units, from the Swedish scientist of that name. Only those rays of the sun, our chief source of radiant energy, which come between 2,900 and 3,200 A.U., can affect our skin. The shortest wavelength in sunlight at the earth's surface, under the best conditions, is about 2,900 A.U. Skin sensitivity decreases with wavelengths longer than

3,000 A.U., and those longer than 3,200 A.U. leave virtually no effect. Ordinarily, sunburn-producing radiation reaches the skin indirectly, and is greatly influenced by the season, the hour of the day, latitude, the clearness of the sky, fog, smoke, and reflections from surrounding water, sand or snow.

Physiologically, the primary changes in the skin are confined to the upper layers or epidermis, which is injured by the action of ultraviolet on the cell proteins and nucleic acids. The resultant liberation of the chemical histamine into the circulation, produces the erythema (reddening) effect so readily noticeable after exposure. There is little, if any, direct action on the blood vessels. Erythema persists a few days, and then changes over to a tan color, due to the appearance of the melanin skin pigment. Depending upon the amount of exposure, and the intensity of the light source, the extent of skin injury may vary from ordinary desquamation (peeling) to the more serious vesiculation. An acute sunburn varies but little from a first-degree burn from any heat source. The lassitude which may follow long exposure to the sun's rays is more apt to be heat stroke, and not due to sunburn.

Doc Silvers says: "Put it down as a hard and fast rule of life that extremes of anything are unhealthful, may be dangerous, and even fatal."

Your natural "built-in" protection from overexposure is derived from the screening action of the outer layer of the skin (stratum corneum). This layer thickens, and the appearance of the melanin pigment is Nature's means of affording you extra protection. Artificially, the best protection is obtained by glass screening or compounds like para-amino-benzoic acid and other chemicals applied to the skin, which are found in all good suntan lotions.

how sunbathing can help and hurt you

The quantitative degree of your susceptibility to sunlight may be observed by the smallest amount of ultraviolet irradiation that will produce reddening of the skin. The erythema threshold varies widely amongst us, and in each of us, at different times. This is due to the thickness of the outer layers of the skin, the condition of the cutaneous blood vessels, the dryness of the skin, and your particular sensitivity to light. Therefore, your own susceptibility to sunlight can only be determined by self-experimentation. So take it easy, be cautious, and follow the instructions for sunbathing given later on.

The good to be obtained from exposure to sunlight is actually indirectly proportional to the degree of sunburn. Therefore, the *less* the sunburn, the *greater* the therapeutic effect. *Always* try to avoid burning your skin, as it will give you the miseries, may do you serious harm, and on top of that, will spoil all your fun. Many a well-intentioned person has ruined his or her vacation by acquiring a severe burn the first day, thereby suffering the tortures of the damned for the rest of the period. Most folks have one vacation a year, usually of two-weeks' duration. If you inadvertently ruin it with sunburn, it will have an adverse effect on your health for an extended period thereafter, and it may well be months before you are really back on your feet and feel like your old self again. So keep in mind that the salutary effects of sunlight are best obtained by *gradual* exposure and the stimulation of your own protective mechanism.

Doc Silvers says: "*Always* help Nature; *never* hinder her. You'll enjoy life's pleasures all the more, and live longer, too."

avoid sunburn of the eyes

Sunburn of the eyes may affect the conjunctiva (white) and the cornea (colored) parts of the eyes, and, like sunburn of the skin, is the result of long exposure to bright sunlight, its reflection, or from other sources of intense light. While uncommon in temperate climates, it frequently occurs after prolonged exposure in snow-covered terrain. This snow blindness is often encountered among explorers who make long treks over the tundras of the arctic or antarctic. Acute photophobia (pain in the eye) is the most prominent symptom. A similar form of eye burn may result from exposure to a welding arc, and has also been attributed to a flash of lightning. Imagine what would happen to our unprotected eyes if we were exposed, even at an otherwise safe distance, to an exploding hydrogen bomb. The flash alone would blind us instantaneously. Many have suffered "eye damage" just from observing a total eclipse of the sun without proper protection at the crucial moment of intense light after darkness.

Protection from eye sunburn is obviously simple, and needs no Rx from me. However, I would caution you strongly against the wearing of dark glasses of the sort obtainable at counters in variety and drug stores. They may be injurious in several ways:

A) Not dark enough to be protective.

B) Too dark, thus reducing the clarity of your vision, and making you subject to bumps and falls.

C) Frames ill-fitting because they are not of the proper size.

D) If you wear glasses for the correction of your vision, ordinary dark glasses won't do unless you use the type which fit over your regular lenses, which are a nuisance to put on and take off.

For some years, dark glasses have been the vogue, and today practically everybody wears them, usually all day long, in winter as well as summer. This is downright silly. It can also be the cause of accidents since eyeglass frames obstruct and limit the area of vision. So if you don't need eyeglasses, don't wear dark glasses except when at the beach, on the water, skiing, and at any other time when sunlight or its reflection may be intense. And even though your eyesight is perfect, get your dark glasses from an optician or optometrist, for even though the lenses have no corrective quality, they will be of the right size and shape for your physiognomy, and the frames will be properly fitted. Should you wear corrective lenses and wish to have dark glasses for appropriate occasions, have them ground to your prescription so that you will be able to see properly while wearing them.

Doc Silvers says: **"This could well be a more cheerful world if all those who wear dark glasses wore rose-colored ones instead."***

using infrared light at home

Skin sensitivity decreases very rapidly as the wave lengths go above 3,000 A.U. But since the skin is more transparent to longer wave lengths, like those of the infrared, they reach the deeper structures of the body, and the physiologic effect is different. Longer wave lengths heat the skin which, in turn, enhances the chemical action of radiant energy, causing marked dilation of the underlying blood vessels. This, you will recollect, is the same effect as that obtained from heat applied with moist compresses.

Infrared, which is at the opposite end of the sun's spectrum, has the longest wave length. It is much more penetrating, and has a more soothing effect upon the skin and deeper tissues than ultraviolet light. Being all heat and little light, infrared produces direct dilatation of the deeper blood vessels, increasing the flow and volume of blood as it courses through the skin and various organs of the body. In this manner, it hastens the absorption of the products of inflammation and relieves swelling and pain following injury.

As with moist heat, infrared should never be used at the outset of an injury. While in the acute stage, cold is first applied, as described previously. Always wait for the subacute stage, usually 48 hours, before making use of the more potent effect of the infrared.

Dry heat may be applied by contact with a hot water bottle or an electric pad. When I was a youngster, mothers frequently used a hot flatiron or a brick heated in the oven and wrapped in a turkish towel to avoid burns. Today, the infrared lamp is more convenient to use, produces even heat over any desired period, and is safer as it does not come in contact with the skin. Use as directed in the instructions that come with the bulb. It provides the same beneficial therapy as moist heat, but is more potent, and is used for the same purposes.

how to use home massage effectively

We have seen how hot and cold treatments—perhaps they should be called "temperature therapy"—are used for various aches and injuries. There is another form of treatment often used in combination with them: massage. When you have a pain of any kind, you instinctively rub it, just as your prehistoric ancestors did a million or more years ago. And in most cases, the pain is relieved, at least to some extent.

Massage, using natural means, is a form of physical medicine commonly applied. While today there are various types of massaging devices, the best mechanism for this purpose is still the human hand. It is more flexible and can be more readily controlled than any apparatus. When properly used, it has a soothing, hypnotic effect, and is beneficial psychologically.

In the case of serious disease or injury, massage, when indicated, must, of course, be used only by a physician or a qualified masseur operating under a doctor's direction. There are, however, many instances of minor maladies which can be treated at home with massage by the layman. In some instances, self-massage can be used, such as rubbing an arm or leg, the forehead, or any other accessible part of the body. Here, for example, is a common complaint which you can take care of yourself.

muscle cramp

A sudden muscle spasm, which commonly occurs in the lower extremities, is excruciatingly painful. It may be due to an awkward, uncomfortable posture which is maintained for some time. A cramp frequently occurs at night. Exposure to cold, dampness, fatigue, or debility tend to such seizures. The rheumatic and gouty also may suffer from them. A spasm lasts from a few seconds to several minutes.

Home Rx:

First stretch the limb with a quick jerk, and it may knock out the cramp. If not, rub the affected place strongly with a quick motion for a minute or two. Should there still be some pain, apply the most convenient form of moist or dry heat.

Except for this and a few other instances, massage is best performed upon the afflicted person by someone else, and there are several good reasons why:

A) The patient can be at rest while the massaging is in progress.

B) The operator can massage parts which are inaccessible to the patient.

C) The patient's attention can be wholly directed to guiding the operator as to the locale, the amount of pressure, and the resultant degree of relief.

D) A soothing feeling is obtained from the touch of the operator's hands which, as it is continued, is hypnotic in its effect.

E) In home massage, the operator is usually the spouse, or some other member of the family in whom the patient places his or her complete confidence and trust. This personal relationship is psychologically beneficial.

The best relief for painful spastic muscles is heat and massage. The advantages of manual massage over mechanical massage are manifested in the physiologic effects of the human touch, an increase in the temperature of the parts under manipulation, better accessibility to the head, neck, and joints, and for its sedative and hypnotic effect upon sensitive tissues.

Massage has a number of very beneficial functions. It stimulates the blood and lymph flow, bringing an increased supply to the surface, reduces the swelling and thickening of tissues, breaks down adhesions, improves nutrition by an increased flow of blood, and aids the functions of the skin in the removal of waste matter. The application of pressure by human touch relieves pain, removes the products of inflammation, and so reduces the irritability of the nerves. Your aches and pains are thereby alleviated, the throbbing which ran you ragged is soon gone, and you are left with that glorious feeling of well-being and elation called euphoria.

The physical therapy which doctors call by the fancy name of massotherapy is broadly divided into five types of manual application.

1. Effleurage

This massage consists of a light stroking movement performed with either one or both hands. The effect is to act on the nerves of the skin and the superficial vessels, thus aiding the circulation and glandular activity. The local congestion is relieved by the touch of the stroking hand at a slow rate, with contact and pressure as light as possible. The response to effleurage is a soothing feeling, the shrinking of skin capillaries, a reduction in skin and body temperature, and the relief of pain. **This light type of massage is indicated particularly for muscle spasms and sprains. When applied over the spinal column and the forehead, it has a beneficial effect for simple headaches and insomnia.** Apply the light stroking for fifteen to twenty minutes, and the *pain* will be relieved.

Applying Effleurage
1) Place the cushions of the tips of the fingers of one hand slightly below the area to be massaged.
2) With only slight pressure, make a long stroke up to, but not over, the affected part.
3) Without pressure, glide the fingers back over the skin to the starting position.
4) Do not lift the fingers from the patient's body throughout the treatment.
5) Repeat until the whole surrounding area has been massaged.

2. Petrissage
Kneading is the most common form of deep massage, and consists of the alternating application and release of pressure on the muscles being treated. Pressure is applied with fingers and thumbs, hand and underlying bone, without moving the hand over the skin. In superficial kneading, pulling the skin up with the thumb and first two fingers, the effect is confined almost exclusively to the skin. Deep kneading involves the muscles beneath the skin, the pressure being increased, and the vessels reduced in diameter by stretching. The result is the stimulation of the vital activities of the tissues being treated, promotion of circulation in the normal direction, and by the reflex effect resulting in the dilation of the blood vessels. **This technique is best used for poor circulation and the breaking down and removal of inflammatory matter (exudates).**

Petrissage is excellent treatment for sprains and fractures, rheumatism of the muscles and joints, and for the relief of constipation.

Applying Petrissage

1) When treating a small area, as in the hand, pick up the flesh between the thumb and fingers.

2) Keep the thumb rigid, and roll the flesh against it with the fingers.

3) Then keep the fingers rigid, and roll the flesh against them with the thumb.

4) Alternate these movements rhythmically a half-dozen times.

5) Then move the hand slightly and repeat the process until the entire affected area has been massaged.

6) In treating a large area, as on the arm or leg, grasp the flesh with the whole of both hands.

7) Keep the fingers steady, and work the thumbs and palms against them in the rolling motion.

8) Repeat a half-dozen times, and then move to another area.

9) Continue for about 15 minutes until the entire area being treated has been massaged.

3. Friction

Friction in massage consists of stroking accompanied by pressure, which has a mechanical effect in emptying the blood and lymph vessels, thus promoting circulation. It also has a reflex action through the stimulation of circulation. **Friction is indicated to stimulate peripheral (outer) circulation, remove fluids which have accumulated in disease, and to reduce swelling and inflammation.** The circulatory stimulation also increases the rate of metabolism thus helping to build up weakened or spastic muscles. Friction consists of rubbing the muscles without picking them up from the bone.

Applying Friction

1) Place the cushions of both thumbs on a spot in the area to be treated.

2) Using slight pressure, massage the underlying tissues by making small circles with the thumbs.

3) Repeat the movement a half-dozen times.

4) Move the thumbs to an adjacent area, and repeat the massage.

5) Continue for about 15 minutes until the whole affected part has been treated.

4. Vibration

Vibratory massage is applied along the course of nerves to sooth them and relax the muscles. This form of massage is readily mastered by the novice and, after a little practice, can be put to good use by any family as it has a most salutary effect in soothing and relaxing the patient.

Applying Vibration

1) With the fingertips lightly drawn together, place them over a nerve. Use one or both hands, as preferred.

2) Keeping the wrist limp, move the fingers quickly up and down in short, shaky movements, thus producing a rapid vibration which passes from the operator to the patient.

3) Keep the movements fast and even as the fingers slowly progress along the course of the nerve.

4) Continue this vibratory massage for a few minutes until the patient expresses relief.

5. Tapotement

Tapotement produces a powerful reflex action on the skin and deeper tissues, thus creating a marked increase in circulation. It is particularly beneficial for the reflex stimulation of the deeper or internal organs.

Applying Tapotement

1) Use one hand for a small area, both hands for a larger one.

2) Close the fist and lightly pound the muscle with the inside edge below the little finger.

3) When using both fists, strike alternately with each one.

4) Go backwards and forwards until the whole area has been covered.

5) Continue for about three minutes.

Massage is an ancient art, having been used in the Orient for 5,000 years and more. The Japanese are particularly expert in massage therapy, though today there are excellent practitioners in other countries as well, particularly the Scandinavian. If you want to experience the wonderful feeling of euphoria obtainable from massage, visit a licensed masseur. Meanwhile, practice the five basic variations of manual massage in your own home, as directed, and you will obtain relief from many of the aches and pains which plague most of us.

Nude Bathing
for Good Health
and Healthy Skin

4   The skin, the organ covering the largest area of the body, has two basic functions. The obvious one is protection of the underlying tissues from disease and injury. The other important purpose is as an aid in the regulation of body temperature. Since they operate automatically, modern man pays little attention to these two organic functions. Instead, the interest is primarily focused on the cosmetic appeal of this enveloping sheath. Everyone desires a clear skin and a good complexion.

The air you breathe, the type of clothing you wear, the moisture in your home and office or shop, and its ventilation, the exercise you take and, of primary importance, how much of your body is exposed to sun and air, are all determining factors in the health and appearance of your skin. A truly healthy skin needs the exposure that all wild life, and even our domesticated animals and pets, have much of the time.

Whether or not one may bathe in the nude depends upon the particular environment, social customs, and the law. On an ocean voyage, for example, it is customary to take a morning constitutional by walking around the ship several times on the promenade deck. If one were to do so stripped to the buff, the offending passenger would be quickly put in irons and confined in the brig. But a daily constitutional while on a sea voyage would be much more beneficial if it could be done in the nude. However, it is not permissible in our society. Even on cruises, bathing attire is only allowed in certain sections of the ship. And on public beaches, local ordinances restrict the degree of epidermic exposure.

I am reminded of the case of a patient who, some 30 years ago, consulted me about a spreading rash on his lower abdomen. I sent him to a dermatologist, who diagnosed the condition as pityriasis rosea, caused by a vegetable fungus. He gave the patient a sun-lamp treatment, and then advised him as follows: "It is summer, and you say that you are going on your vacation. So why pay me for sunlamp therapy when all you need do is expose the affected area to the sun?"

This man spent his vacations at Long Beach on the south shore of Long Island. In those days, local ordinance required the wear-ing of two-piece bathing suits for male bathers, and a police officer patrolled the boardwalk above the beach to enforce the regulation. So, while his fiancée kept an eye out for the cop, my patient re-moved the top of his bathing suit, and pushed down his trunks so that the rash would be exposed to the healing rays of Old Sol. Whenever the police officer approached, he would hurriedly pull up his trunks, and slip into his bathing shirt. However, one day when his sweetheart was not there to keep a lookout, he was ap-prehended by the cop, arrested, and fined. Therefore, although he was staying at a fine beach resort on the Atlantic, he was forced to purchase a sunlamp and treat himself indoors. This, to my mind, is absolutely senseless.

Today, trunks are considered sufficient male bathing attire in the U.S., which is some indication of progress. But the bikini for women is generally taboo, though permitted at resorts in Europe and elsewhere. Nude bathing—among both sexes—is acceptable in the Scandinavian countries and in Russia. But we are so hypocritical about nudity and sex in this country that it will be many a long day —if ever—before bathing in the all-together, except for certain care-fully regulated nudist colonies, will be permitted in America. Our social heritage is so deep-seated that progress is infinitely slower than the peregrinations of an aged tortoise.

nudity isn't shameful

Hardly 50 years ago—if you are of my generation, you will remember; if you are of the so-called "modern" generation, you can ask your grandparents—women didn't bathe in the nude, even in the privacy of their own bathroom! In preparing to take a bath, a female of that day first disrobed in the bedroom, and put on a cotton, full-length nightgown. Then she entered the bathroom, closed the door, and locked it, perhaps adding a padlock for double security. The tub having been filled with water of the desired temperature, she stepped into it, and gently seated herself—without removing the nightgown! Lifting the gown no more than necessary, she soaped and scrubbed herself underneath it, thus avoiding the embarrassment of seeing her own naked body. Standing up, she took a large sponge and rinsed herself off as best she could. Then getting out of the tub, she dried herself with a Turkish towel and, wrapping it around her, finally removed the wet nightgown.

This sterile method of taking a bath goes back thousands of years, and was rooted in the tradition that it is sinful for a woman to view her own genitalia. Vestiges of this silly custom may be found to this very day. In the hinterlands of the U.S., and in other "civilized" countries, women still carry on this practice. There are traces of it even among the most sophisticated women. Nurses have a standard joke about women who consult a general practitioner or gynecologist about a genital disorder. When they are asked where their trouble lies, they invariably blush, lower their eyes, and whisper: "Down there."

Physicians—like artists, sculptors, and photographers, who portray the unadorned figure—are inured to the exposure of complete nudity, male or female, however perfect the physique. But only rarely does a doctor encounter a female patient who is not hesitant about disrobing, even though the nurse provides her with a shapeless gown to wear during the examination. In contrast, I am reminded of an experience which occurred in my early days as a G. P.

One morning I received a phone call from a regular patient who asked if I would stop by to attend her younger sister, who was running a temp. Mrs. Alice was married to a Wall Street man who traveled extensively. They had two sons, who went to private school, and were away at camp all summer. Under these circumstances, to avoid loneliness, Alice had arranged to have her younger sister Betty live with her, as their parents were deceased.

Shortly after receiving the call, I drove over to the address in my ancient jalopy. I rang the apartment bell and Alice promptly opened the door. She greeted me and directed me to her sister's bedroom. I started toward it, and then suddenly stopped dead in my tracks as I belatedly realized that Mrs. Alice was as naked as Eve! The only thing that avoided complete nudity was a large scrubbing brush which she held in a strategic position.

"I must apologize, Doctor," she began.

"Oh, that's quite all right," I said nonchalantly, thinking she was making an excuse for her lack of attire. But I was mistaken about her intention.

"I'm sorry," she explained, "that you came just as I was in the midst of scrubbing the floors. They're wet, so be careful you don't slip."

I wrote out a prescription for her sister and, as I prepared to leave, Mrs. Alice was dressed, ready to go to the drugstore.

"Frankly," I observed with a smile, "I was rather surprised when you opened the door to let me in. I've been practicing for less than two years, and though I've cut up cadavers and delivered babies during my interneship, I'm afraid that I'm not yet quite conditioned to the sights a veteran physician takes as a matter of course."

"When my sister and I do heavy housework," she explained with a laugh, "scrubbing floors like today, washing the walls, or painting, we work without clothes. Wearing something interferes with our chores, and the clothes get all messed up and have to be washed. So we avoid all that, and get the work done more easily and faster. Afterwards, we soak in a hot tub, and then take a refreshing cool shower. We're from the Old Country—Finland, to be exact—and we learned this custom from our mothers and grandmothers."

"A healthful habit it is," I said as I left, "and I wish that more of my patients would observe it."

"Thank you, Doctor," Mrs. Alice replied. "And, the next time you call, I'll make sure to be dressed, as I wouldn't want to shock our family physician."

Doc Silvers says: "The only unwholesome aspect about nudity is being ashamed of it."

Adam and Eve were unconscious of their nudity while they lived in the Garden of Eden. But then they ate of the forbidden fruit, and, as related in Genesis 3:7, "And the eyes of them both were opened, and they knew that they were naked; and they sewed fig leaves together, and made themselves aprons." Today the fashion industry is still sewing fig leaves to cover up milady's most beautiful attributes.

I am not, mind you, advocating nudism as a cult. That is a social attitude which may, or may not, appeal to you. What you do about it is your own private business, and none of my concern. My sole purpose here is to acquaint you with the inestimable value of nudity as a wholesome and healthful therapy.

Keep in mind that all parts of the body benefit from exposure to the benign elements. So when, outside the privacy of your own home, you bathe in water, sun, or air, wear as little as the law will allow in order to obtain maximum exposure. Don't get into trouble, as my Long Beach patient did. Before going to a strange resort, ask your travel agent what bathing costumes are permitted, or refer to a guidebook. And if the opportunity ever does present itself to bathe in the nude without incurring the wrath of the local constabulary, by all means try it. If you have never done so before, you will discover that, however scant your bathing attire, taking it off and dipping into the ocean or a mountain lake is a refreshingly new and exhilarating experience.

the benefits of artificial sunlight

Despite my emphasis on the therapeutic values of nudity, some may well say that their own particular environment does not make it convenient or permissible, and I appreciate their position. None of my patients has ever been incarcerated for so-called "indecent exposure," and I wouldn't want any of my readers to get into that predicament, either. If one of them should, I unfortunately couldn't be of any assistance as I do not know any friendly judges. So unless nudism is a cult with you, and you stand ready to back its philosophy, whatever the consequences, please stay out of the jailhouse.

Happily, there is a way by which you can circumvent the dictum of society, and enjoy nude sun bathing in your home without incurring the wrath of the law. All you need do is make a health investment in a sunlamp. The mercury-vapor quartz lamp, the older carbon arc lamp, and a number of others, deliver ultraviolet rays. While they are not, of course, equal in quantity and effect to noonday sunlight in clear weather, the end result from exposure to the ultraviolet rays from the lamp is the same as that from the natural source, and the liberation of Vitamin D from the ergosterol in the skin is also comparable. There is the danger of overexposure, just as with sunlight, but I have no hesitation in assuming that my intelligent readers will carefully follow the directions which come with the unit, thereby avoiding all harm.

how to select and use a sunlamp properly

In selecting a sunlamp, you will find that there are many varieties, from just a bulb, which can be screwed into any light socket, to more elaborate units. Prices range from about $10 to around $50. If the device does not include a timer, obtain a kitchen or darkroom timer. Never expose yourself to the lamp without first setting the timer to the number of minutes recommended in the instructions. Always wear dark goggles, which usually come with the unit, and protect your lips with vaseline or cold cream.

Irradiation is used by dermatologists for almost every type of rash of the skin. Ultraviolet rays are beneficial in stimulating glandular functions which have an indirect effect on the skin. Absorption of Vitamin D is essential for the proper functioning of the little gland on top of the thyroid, called the parathyroid. It is the chief regulator of your calcium metabolism, and determines how much of this essential mineral your blood serum can absorb and retain. Without the optimal amount of calcium in your blood serum, bathing all of the muscle and nerve junctions, you become tense and the muscles go into spasm. And remember that you must consume enough dairy foods and leafy greens to supply the grist for your calcium mill.

Ultraviolet irradiation is also valuable in treating acne vulgaris, the common pimples from which many teen-agers suffer, psoriasis, the scaly, shimmering rash usually occurring on the backs of the elbows and the front of the knees, and lupus vulgaris, a form of tuberculosis of the skin. It has little if any value in furunculosis (multiple boils) and other pus-forming and fungus infections. There are some skin diseases where sun rays are contraindicated, so all the above require the attention and supervision of a physician. Your purpose in using a sunlamp is in the cosmetic treatment of your skin, giving it an attractive light tan, helping to keep it clear, and for the acquisition of Vitamin D.

Sunlamps are customarily purchased for winter use. However, they can be used, upon occasion, in summer as well, on rainy days, and when you don't have the opportunity to get out in the sun. They can also be used to tan the parts of the body (always keep the loins protected) which are covered by your swimsuit when outdoors, thus obtaining an even, all-over tan. If you have a pale, sallow complexion, and your vocation requires you to be indoors most of the time, use a sunlamp on your face for a few minutes—being sure to wear the proper dark glasses—three times a week for that attractive outdoorsy look.

give your skin the nutrition it needs

A popular slang expression, referring to eating, runs like this: "I'm going to feed my face." Interestingly and amusingly enough, there's more than a grain of truth in it for, if you want to have good skin, that is literally what you must do: "Feed your face."

The condition of your skin depends, in large measure, on good nutrition. If you eat properly, adequately, and your diet is well balanced, your skin will benefit thereby. Every animal lover knows that the coat of his pet is conditioned by the variety and value of the vitamins and minerals in the food which it is fed.

For a clear and healthy skin, you need the aid of nutritive oils.

The oils taken internally carry the vitamins which are fat soluble, namely, A, D, K, and E. These are all essential to a healthy, smooth, and elastic skin.

The best of the oils, and very likely the oldest in use by man, is still cod liver oil. It is rich, not only in polyunsaturates, but in Vitamins A and D. The liver oil of fish from the sea is an excellent source of iodine, and you can get your normal requirement by taking one ounce (2 tablespoons) daily.

The traditional and most ancient oil in use for cooking and salads is olive oil. Italians and other nationalities still prefer it, and it is unquestionably an excellent oil for cooking and other purposes. Today, however, it is expensive in comparison with the other vegetable oils now readily available. Corn oil, cotton seed oil, peanut oil, and even sesame oil, are all every bit as nutritious and easily digestible as olive oil; but if, despite its relatively higher cost, you prefer the latter, by all means continue to use it.

Doc Silvers says: "**By feeding your skin from the inside while tanning yourself on the outside, you have the very best therapy for healthy skin and an attractive complexion.**"

Bathing Remedies to
Get Lasting Results

5 There are five general types of natural bathing therapy. Let us examine them in detail so that you will appreciate their value, and be able to make the best use of them.

gain these big benefits of water therapy

Hydrotherapy, or treatment by the use of water, is of great value in the maintenance and prolongation of health. In bathing, the skin organ acts as a transmitter of any stimuli which may be applied to its surface. In this process, an exchange of molecules occurs between the water and the skin tissue, which alters its structure. This external stimulation of the skin in bathing directly influences the delicate balance of the sympathetic nervous system. In that way, the tensions of the body are definitely controlled.

Many ailments result from the failure of the skin to adapt itself to changes in temperature, natural or artificial. Thus if the normal functional activity of the skin is improved so that it can better withstand changes in temperature, there is substantially less chance of illness. This is hydrotherapy's principal purpose. In addition to being used as a curative measure, it reinforces the resources of the skin, reducing sensitivity to external changes, and building up greater resistance to disease. Since temperature is the main force in hydrotherapy, water is classified in degrees in this way:

A) Cold—below 70 degrees F. Stimulating effect.
B) Tepid—70 to 98 degrees F. Comforting effect.
C) Hot—above 98 degrees F. Sedative effect.

how to use cold-water therapy

In cold-water bathing, the peripheral blood vessels first contract, and later normally dilate. This action and reaction has a favorable effect in improving circulation. However, if the cold is not sufficiently intense, the vessels do not develop secondary dilation and, as a result, the feeling of well-being will not occur. In addition, if the bath is of too long a duration, the veins become congested, and normal circulation is impeded. The skin must be in a healthy state to react properly to any form of stimulation. The difficulty lies in the fact that the capacity to react to the stimulus of water varies with each individual. This is principally because we are constantly attired in confining clothes which prevent the skin from reacting favorably to external influences and, in time, dull its normal response to them. To find your own individual reaction, do this:

Home Rx:

1) Using a bath thermometer, regulate the temperature of the water for a cold bath or shower to approximately 68 degrees F.

2) Stay in it for three minutes, no more.

3) If the normal feeling of euphoria does not result, the next time bathe for five minutes at the same water temperature.

4) Should this not prove effective, reduce the temperature of the water to a little above 60 degrees F. and bathe for three minutes.

5) If this still doesn't work, bathe for five minutes at the colder temperature.

One of these methods will provide the most favorable reaction for your particular constitution, and you will thoroughly enjoy the stimulation of cold tub or shower bathing thereafter.

There is nothing quite like the lift one gets from cold-water bathing, whether at home or outdoors. There are just a few simple precautions, which should always be observed.

A) Don't take a cold bath shortly after a heavy meal. Wait an hour or more.

B) Warm up with a little mild exercise before taking a cold bath.

C) Never plunge into a cold tub or dash under a cold shower.

D) In case of a tub bath, step in and pat the cold water on your legs. Do the same with your arms. Don't immerse yourself completely until then.

E) For a cold shower, pat water on your arms and legs, your chest, and the back of your neck, before stepping under the direct spray.

There are several important contraindications to cold-water bathing:

1) Don't when the body is chilled by the onstart of a fever.

2) Don't when you feel abnormally weak or debilitated.

3) Don't if you are elderly and unaccustomed to an active life.

4) Don't if you suffer from a heart ailment or circulatory condition, unless your physician approves.

Otherwise, if you are in normally good health, enjoy cold water bathing, both indoors and outdoors. Don't be afraid of cold, whether it be water or air. In earlier days, the American Indian wore a minimum of clothing, even during the harsh New England winters. It did him no harm—in fact, it did him a lot of good—and he didn't mind the extreme cold, as evidenced by this story:

> "How is it that you wear only a loin cloth," inquired an astonished white man, "when it is snowing today?"
> "Your face covered?" the Indian asked.
> "Why, no," the white man said. "But what has that got to do with it?"
> "Me all face," the Indian stoically replied.

Doc Silvers says: "Mark Twain said that 'Clothes make the man.' But it is largely the lack of them that keeps him healthy."

how to use hot-water therapy

There are three principal purposes for taking a hot bath.

1) To induce sweating, which eliminates waste matter through

the pores of the skin. As everyone knows, there is nothing so cleansing as a good soaping and scrubbing in a hot bath, either tub or shower, followed by a rinse.

2) To bring on a feeling of comfort and relaxation. Being sedative in effect, it acts as a tranquilizer and, as I point out in the chapter on sleep, thus obviates the need for drugs.

3) After vigorous exercise, a hot bath, followed by a cold rinse, is effective in preventing the stiffness which ordinarily results from muscular activity. It is especially helpful if you have participated in a sport or game which you do not play regularly.

A Spa Bath at Home

Balneotherapy or spa bathing has benefited mankind since ancient times. To this day, those who can afford it, travel to various famous spas in this country and abroad. However, if you haven't the time or money for an extensive—and expensive!—visit to a spa, you can enjoy the equivalent of spa bathing right in your own tub. Here is my original prescription for a therapeutic bath which is similar in its beneficial effects to the best of spa therapy. All of the ingredients are readily obtainable, and inexpensive.

Home Rx:

Epsom salt	4 oz. or 8 tablespoons
Bicarbonate of soda	1 oz. or 2 tablespoons
Oil of wintergreen	30 drops or ½ teaspoon
Alpha keri	½ oz. or 1 tablespoon
(Westwood Pharmaceuticals)	

Mix the above ingredients thoroughly in enough water at 103 degrees F. to cover the body above the shoulders. Remain immersed for 20 minutes. Keep your head out of the water, and avoid wetting the eyes. While oil of wintergreen is irritating to mucous membranes, the alpha keri, which is an excellent emulsifier, disperses the wintergreen oil, and so avoids accidental irritation of sensitive parts. If you find that your skin is sensitive to the oil, reduce the amount the next time from 30 to 20 drops. Because of the oil, the bottom of the tub may be a bit slippery, so use care when getting out. Don't dry yourself with a towel as it is advantageous to have the healthful ingredients remain on the skin. Instead, air-dry yourself with mild exercise or by just moving around.

This soothing spa bath is muscle relaxing, and makes the skin softer and more pliable. The treatment also relieves itching, dryness, and most mild skin irritations. Its effects are ideal when taken just before bedtime, making it easy to sleep.

Hot Packs for Relief of Pain

For the relief of pain in muscles or joints, one of the best wet hot packs is simply prepared with flaxseed. Fill a small cloth bag, about six inches square, with the seed, and sew up the opening. Steep it in very hot water for several minutes. When cool enough to touch on the back of the hand, apply to the painful area. Keep it on for one hour, then wait an hour before the next application. Use as often as needed. This flaxseed poultice holds the heat longer than any other form of hot pack.

why you should water the tree of life

Our feet and legs are analogous to the roots of a tree, which hold up the torso or trunk. They support the skeleton and the weight of the whole body. The sap—the blood, that is—travels down through the arteries and is driven back up to the heart and lungs via the veins. Because of their strategic position, the feet perform a very important function in maintaining good health. It will be found, therefore, that a hot foot bath has many beneficial therapeutic effects.

Home Rx:

1) Pour water at about body temperature (98.6 degrees F.) into a deep basin. If you don't have one that is large enough, put a stool in the bathtub, or use one of the fitted seats made for the purpose. Never sit on the edge of the tub as you may slip and injure yourself.

2) With your feet in the basin or tub, add water until it reaches halfway up your legs, about the middle of the calf.

3) Add hot water slowly, gradually increasing the temperature to the limit of tolerance, usually under 115 degrees F.

4) Soak your feet and legs for about 15 minutes, or until the water starts to cool off.

5) Remove your legs from the bath, and rub them with a washcloth rinsed in cold water.

6) Omit number 5 if it is desirable to have the dilatation of the blood vessels last as long as possible.

This foot bath of increasing temperature produces an improvement in the surface circulation of the extremities immersed, and also has a definite beneficial effect on the heart muscle. It, therefore, has great value in improving circulation; hence it may be prescribed for moderate heart conditions. In cases of high blood pressure, with its accompanying headache and resultant insomnia, the hot foot bath often provides great relief. Its effect is most favorable in chronic bronchitis, bronchial asthma, bladder irritations, intestinal disturbance, and many of the common respiratory infections. Finally, if your feet ache, and you are tired and out of sorts, you will find this hot foot bath "just what the doctor ordered."

effective salt water bathing at home

Salt water has a very stimulating effect, as you know if you are accustomed to ocean bathing. However, those of us who live in the northern states have this opportunity in our own localities for only about ten weeks in the year. But in the colder months, we can take invigorating salt baths in our own tubs. And though sun and air are not available, the bath itself is an effective therapeutic measure.

Home Rx:

1) First take a vessel whose capacity you know, and roughly estimate the amount of water you usually use when having a tub bath.

2) Get sea salt at a health food store or drugstore, or use common table salt, iodized preferred.

3) If you don't have a bath thermometer, purchase a good make. Every home should have one as the temperature of the water is the most influential factor in tub bathing.

4) For simulated ocean bathing, have the water temperature at about 68 degrees F.

5) Add one pound of salt for each ten gallons of water, which approximates the brine content of the sea, about 3%.

6) Stir thoroughly until the salt is dissolved.

7) Immerse yourself slowly, especially if you are warm, first the feet, then the hands and arms, before sitting down.

8) Lave your body, with the exception of the face and head (don't get the salt water in your eyes) for 15 minutes or so, when you will feel greatly stimulated and refreshed.

how ocean bathing can pay big dividends

The three principal factors involved in bathing at the seashore, each complex in itself, are water, air, and sun. The special attributes of sea air are freedom from dirt and dust, higher barometric pressure, and greater oxygen content. A sea breeze—which acts as a natural air-conditioning mechanism—purifies the air, spreading warmth evenly and maintaining an agreeable degree of humidity.

The sun's rays are intensified by the reflection of radiation from water and sand. While humidity does not diminish biologically important wave lengths, the infrared are absorbed, thus making solar radiation at the shore relatively cooler than at higher altitudes.

Contrary to popular opinion, the body cannot absorb any minerals from sea water, no matter how long the period of immersion. However, ocean bathing has many definite effects, which are attributed to the following factors:

A) Air temperature.

B) Water temperature.

C) The difference between the temperature of your skin and that of the water.

D) Humidity.

E) Barometric pressure.

F) Intensity of sunlight.

G) Wind velocity.

H) The irritating effect of the salt in the water on the skin.

I) The stimulating effect of the breaking waves.

All of these, not only alone but in their relation to each other, determine the end result of your sojourn at the seashore. In addition—and most important of all—is the degree of efficiency of the heat regulatory powers of your particular constitution. Due to modern heating, and the excess of clothing worn during most of the day, your skin loses its natural ability to adjust to sudden temperature changes, which are normally accomplished by the tonic contraction of the blood vessels. The biologic effects of climate on your constitution depend primarily on your heat-absorbing capacity, which is in turn influenced by temperature, humidity, barometric pressure, wind, and intensity of the sunshine. Fortunately, at the bathing beaches, where we are permitted comparative nudity in our attire, the skin soon becomes acclimated, and the natural heat regulatory function is readily regained. The mucous membranes also transmit the effects of climatic change and influence the glands of internal secretion, as well as the blood vessels and the independent nervous system. This is only temporary, however, for when we go back to our "civilized" way of urban life, with its lack of exposure to air and sunshine, the body's natural "thermostat" loses its sensitivity again.

using climatotherapy for better health

Climatotherapy is planned exposure to an atmosphere with a heat-arbsorbing capacity different from that of our normal home and work surroundings, which is reinforced by the proper application of the natural elements: water, air, and sun. Each of us has a "comfort zone" in which we do not perspire, and are not chilled, because our production of body heat is in equilibrium with the heat-absorbing capacity of our environment. If your heat-absorbing capacity is greater than that of your surroundings, the resultant effect will be stimulating. On the other hand, if it should be less heat-absorbing, it will have a sedative effect upon you.

Biologically, a stimulating climate conserves and produces heat because of a heightened tone of the skin blood vessels, and an elevation of the rate at which you can burn up oxygen. Just the reverse is triggered by a sedative climate. There is greater relaxation of the control of the blood vessels, and bodily activity, and the basal metabolic rate is consequently lowered. To emphasize the significance of metabolism to those who may not appreciate its importance, may I say that it is a term applied to the building up and breaking down of billions of cellular structures, a constant process which sustains growth and life. Basal metabolism indicates the amount of oxygen required for tissue change essential to carry on life in a state of complete rest.

are you "discomfortable?"

When it is uncomfortably hot, folks often smile wanly while mopping their brow, and facetiously repeat the familiar phrase: "It isn't the heat, it's the humidity." As with many old sayings, there's more than a grain of truth in it. Today we know that discomfort depends, not on temperature or humidity alone, but upon the relationship between them. Just a few years back, meteorologists compiled a new figure to add to their weather reports. At first it was called the Discomfort Index. But soon after it came into use, businessmen rose up in wrath, declaring that it hurt their trade. Stores in metropolitan areas said that women wouldn't go shopping if the weather was said to be discomforting. Resort owners said that, when the DI was high, instead of crowding the beaches, people stayed at home and cooled off with fans or air conditioners.

With all this hue and cry, something had to be done. But just what? The weather couldn't be changed, that's for sure. So, putting their collective heads together, the meteorologists came up with a positively brilliant idea: they changed the name of the index. It's still the same discomforting rating, but now it is called the Temperature-Humidity Index. Here is what it means, as reported in *The New York Times*:

> "The Temperature-Humidity Index tries to describe numerically the human discomfort resulting from the combined effects of temperature and moisture. It is approximated by adding dry bulb and wet bulb temperature readings, multiplying the sum by 0.4 and adding 15. Estimates indicated that in the summer about ten percent of the people will be uncomfortable even before the Index passes 70; and almost everybody would be uncomfortable, many feeling miserable, at 80 or above."

And that's what the THI means to you. If it is 68 or less, you should feel comfortable. When it hits 70, one in ten will experience discomfort. And when it rises to 80 or more, everyone is "discomfortable." Although it is no longer called the Discomfort Index, you can, of course, still use the THI to plan your day. When it hits the 80's, it is best not to leave the house. Instead, keep cool by ocean bathing in your own bathtub. But keep your plans to yourself, for since the term has been changed our businessmen are happy, and we wouldn't want them to get up in arms again.

know how to play it safe

In bathing as a tonic and stimulant, the water must be colder than body temperature. The ideal temperature for outdoor bathing in a temperature climate during the summer months is 68 degrees. There is one rule of primary importance which you should always observe:

Don't stay in the water for more than 20 minutes at a time.

You risk your health—even your life—every time you ignore this basic regulation. Even if you are a "muscle man" or an athletic woman, and an expert swimmer besides, you take a chance of drowning. The patient of mine, previously mentioned, who summered at Long Beach, told me of two friends of his who had a cottage there. They were in their early twenties, muscular and vigorous. Each afternoon, after their day's work in the city was done, they would take the train to Long Beach. Immediately upon arrival, they slipped into their bathing suits, and went out for a swim. One early evening, while my patient watched them from the beach, they plunged into the surf and started swimming out to sea, as usual. The surf can get very rough at Long Beach, and that day it was especially turbulent. The life guard blew his whistle, warning them to come back, but to no avail. Another guard rowed out in an open raft, but by the time he reached their position, they had gone under. Fifteen minutes later, their bodies were brought ashore, and, although long and tireless efforts were made to resuscitate them, they could not be revived. And, mind you, these were strong young men who were proud of their aquatic prowess.

Doc Silvers says: "It is said that, when a person drowns, his whole life passes before him. But it is an expensive movie to see as the price of admission is your life."

So remember, stay in the water not more than 20 minutes. Then come out and rest for an equal length of time. A feeling of comfortable and exhilarating warmth should follow all cold water bathing. If you experience discomfort or chilliness, and your teeth start chattering, don't go in the water again that day.

How to Use the Sun
as a Master Medicine

6 Sun bathing (heliotherapy) is a necessary natural therapeutic for our so-called "civilized" society, which insists upon wearing garments in private, as well as in public, and often even in bed. As a consequence, our bodies are deprived of essential vitamin D, whose main source of supply is the sun. In an attempt to counterbalance this lack of viosterol, we add it to milk, butter and margarine. But still the best way to acquire and absorb it is from Old Sol. And here is the right way to get the most beneficial results without any ill effects:

1) Sunbathe *only* between the hours of eight to ten in the morning, and three to five in the afternoon, on Standard Time. If the place where you bathe is on Daylight Saving Time, deduct one hour from local time.

2) For initial exposure, sunbathe for 15 minutes, and not a minute more. Ten minutes for redheads and the fair-haired as their skin is more sensitive to the sun's rays.

3) If there is no reaction of excessive redness, increase the exposure to 20 minutes the second day.

4) An increase of five minutes each day thereafter is permissible as long as no painful redness results.

5) Even after your skin is nicely tanned, do not bathe in direct sunlight for more than an hour a day.

6) It is wiser not to lie flat on the beach while sunbathing. You will get a more even, all-over tan by being active and moving around.

7) Suntan lotions are of value in preventing sunburn as they cut down exposure to the actinic rays of the sun, thus preventing excessive reddening and blistering of the skin. Paraminobenzoic acid was the first found to provide this protective property. Other chemicals, now being used, are just as effective. Buy any well-known brand which has been time-tested.

The most beautiful tan I ever saw was on two young Italian girls who were sunbathing on a Connecticut beach. They went about getting a glorious tan intelligently and sensibly. Italians use a lot of olive oil in the preparation of meals, and these two sun-bathers, in addition to getting it internallv, were applying it exter-nally. They had selected an isolated section of the beach and, instead of lying down as most sunbathers do, they stood up and leaned against a large rock, constantly turning and moving about to give their entire bodies an even tan. Wanting to get an all-over tan, they wore only the briefest of briefs, and kept towels handy to cover their bosoms when an occasional stroller pased by. They had lovely figures, and when I observed them—I'll admit I took a long look—their natural olive skin had turned to a glowing golden brown.

8) Take a cleaning shower *before* sunbathing as the maximum benefit from absorption of naturally formed Vitamin D is obtained thereby.

9) Do *not* take a shower *after* sunbathing as it removes con-siderable Vitamin D from the skin, much having been found on the rough Turkish towels used for drying the body.

10) If you have been bathing in the water and your skin is still wet, air-dry your body by walking around until you are dry enough to get dressed.

how to get instant relief from insect bites

Outdoor bathing in water, sun and air naturally makes you vulnerable to stings from bees, wasps, and other insects, especially if most of your skin is exposed, which, if you take my advice, it will be. But if you *are* stung, don't get all heated up wildly beating the air in fruitless effort to destroy the attacker. Instead, always keep a small vial of aromatic spirits of ammonia and a little cotton in your bathing kit. As soon as you are bitten, apply a cotton swab saturated with the ammonia to the painful spot. The ammonia neutralizes the acid in the sting and immediately relieves the pain. My many summers as a camp doctor have provided ample proof, as you can well imagine, that this simple antidote works every time.

a dozen ways to beat the heat

1) Eat plenty of high-protein foods: meat, eggs, cheese, as a bulwark against the exhaustion common when active in hot weather.

2) Salt your food liberally (unless otherwise recommended by your physician).

3) Avoid fats and carbohydrates.

4) Never sit down to a large, heavy meal. Have frequent snacks instead.

5) Keep your weight down.

6) Drink lots of liquids: water, milk, coffee, tea, sodas, in that order. Have them cold or hot, as you prefer. Take alcoholic beverages in moderation. They won't cool you off but, if they calm you down, you won't mind the heat so much.

7) Take frequent showers. Start with warm water, and gradually cool it off. Don't dry yourself vigorously with a towel as you will get all heated up again. Instead, pat your body with it or, preferably, air-dry yourself by moving around.

8) While at work, stop and relax for a few minutes every hour.

9) Wear lightweight clothing.

10) Exercise less.

11) Get a good night's sleep.

12) Remember that the coolest and most comfortable sleeping garment is your own skin, which will not irritate you by wrinkles and folds.

air bathing in the nude

The most neglected form of bathing therapy is air bathing. We breathe too cool, air-conditioned air in our offices in the summer, and too warm air in our overheated homes in the winter. We are constantly in some kind of air, and we breathe it all day and all night long. So why, you wonder, does Doc Silvers prescribe bathing in the air ?

Well, as I have emphasized before, and very likely shall again, we keep our bodies so covered up in underclothes, shirts and blouses, pants and skirts, jackets and coats, shoes and stockings, scarves and hats, that we derive little benefit from the air around us. In fact, we live in a hothouse as though we were some exotic plant. No wonder that the skin, which is the largest organ in the body, is unable to carry out its natural and normal functions.

Everyone can get all of the benefits from natural exposure to air and sunshine in the privacy of the home. Air bathing is invigorating even during the winter months in a temperate climate when the sun's rays come at an angle which is no longer capable of producing a skin tan. Forget about the tan which has faded since your summer vacation, and enjoy the therapeutic benefits of cool, moist air on your exposed body.

Home Rx:

1) Select a room and a time of day when the sun shines in the windows.

2) Open the windows since the violet and ultraviolet rays of the sun cannot penetrate glass. (Note to millionaires and wealthy widows: Have the windows made of quartz, which permits entry of the beneficial rays.)

3) Strip to the buff. If the room is so situated that you can be seen from outside, wear a bathing suit to satisfy the prying eyes of the minions of the law. In this connection, please note that, while I prescribe bathing in the complete nude whenever possible, in water, sun, air, and their combination, you also obtain beneficial results when only part of the body is exposed. In fact, sun on half of the skin area produces enough Vitamin D to supply the entire body with its necessary daily requirement of viosterol.

4) Place a large, soft pillow on the sunny area of the floor.

5) Seat yourself comfortably, using a back support, if desired. If you are in a philosophical frame of mind, assume the cross-legged Yogi position and contemplate your navel.

6) Bathe in the sun and air for a half-hour.

7) Remember, as with sunbathing outdoors, do not take a shower afterwards as you will lose much of the viosterol acquired.

8) Take these combination sun-and-air baths indoors, during the winter months, as often as convenient, several times a week, if possible.

9) Don't be concerned if the sun doesn't seem very bright. You will get an adequate dose of Vitamin D, nevertheless, and you'll benefit, too, from the invigorating outdoor air, which is far more refreshing than that of your undoubtedly overheated home. Many research studies over the years have shown that 68 degrees F. is the best temperature for work, exercise, play, and rest.

Doc Silvers says: "Give your skin a chance to do its job by exposing your body to sun and air all the year around."

how climate influences your health

Much has been written and said about the advantages of certain parts of the world for health and longevity. Let us examine the scientific aspect of Climatotherapy, or treatment of the individual by climate, which is just beginning to receive the attention its importance warrants.

In any given region of the world, the amount of energy you will have to expend on work and other activities depends upon your basic energy level, which, you will recollect, is called metabolism. The ease with which you lose body heat determines the energy level at which you can perform your best work. Our bodies are not 100% efficient as energy conversion machines. In fact, only about 25% is put to use. Comparatively speaking, however, that isn't too bad since an automobile engine is only around 20% efficient, 80% of the energy being a total loss. So respect your body, and take good care of it as it is by far a more wonderful mechanism than man himself, despite automation and space ships, can ever hope to create.

All of our vital functions are possible only because of the conversion of energy from the cellular combustion of the food we consume each day. The body is extremely sensitive to the ease with which its waste heat can be thrown off. Therefore, it has less difficulty in the delicate task of energy conversion when it can lose its transferred heat most readily. This is where environmental climate comes in. When it is easy for the body to get rid of its heat, growth is more rapid, maturity comes early, and resistance to infection is higher. In addition, the excess of energy spills over into more positive and dynamic health. On the other hand, as heat loss becomes more difficult, these indices of body vitality become depressed, resulting in a less active, more vegetative form of existence.

Among the principal factors which influence our health, like genetic background and an adequate food supply, the climatic environment has an important place. You may have the proper food supply, according to modern nutritional standards, and yet be unable to utilize it efficiently. With the markedly lowered combustion level of people in tropical lands, more vitamins are needed to properly utilize each gram of food than are required for the optimal response in cooler climes. But though you are less energetic in warmer places, your body is a more efficient working machine, and shows less evidence of mental wear and tear. In cooler or temperate areas, while you are more buoyant and dynamic, there is the danger that you may overeat, and also succumb to the gradual wearing down process resulting from too strenuous an existence.

Even storms, with their accompanying sudden changes in temperature, humidity, and barometric pressure, are now known to be major disturbing factors in regions where turbulent weather is prevalent. Each one of us differs appreciably in our sensitiveness to storm changes. Some may be utterly unfitted for a healthful existence in a stormy region, and would be far better off living in a calmer area. Oldsters in particular, who suffer from degenerative diseases, will feel much better if, upon retirement, they settle in places like the Gulf Coast, Florida, or Southern California. A winter climate is considered sedative when its mean monthly temperature is above 55 degrees F., enabling an all-year outdoor life.

what to do about the weather

"Everybody talks about the weather," and Charles Dudley Warner, "but nobody does anything about it." But something *can* be done about it. John D. Rockefeller, Senior, sent out a group of medical men and scientists to find the most equable place to live in these United States. After thorough and lengthy investigation, a place was selected on the east coast of Florida, about 90 miles south of Jacksonville, a small village now known as Ormond Beach. There it rarely gets too cold in the winter to interfere with a game of golf, or too hot in the summer to keep one off the beach. The elder Rockefeller spent the latter part of his life in this little town and, as you know, he lived into his nineties, despite the fact that he suffered from a chronic stomach ailment for many years. But, you protest, you are not a multimillionaire as Rockefeller was; and neither am I. Still, while we can't change the weather where we are, we can move to a more healthful climate. The early pioneers piled all their worldly possessions into a Conestoga wagon, tossed in the wife and kids, and trekked from the Atlantic Coast all the way to California, and had to fight the Indians along the way. It took them months, but with modern transportation you can make it within a week. So what's stopping you?

All right then, you don't want to leave your old home town, you'd miss Aunt Alice and Uncle Joe, and there's the mighty important matter of earning a living. Today Americans are always on the go; we have, in fact, become a nomadic people. However, if you'd feel happier in your present surroundings, by all means stay there. In that case, while you can't change the weather, you can make the best use of it by following the suggestions in this chapter, which, to sum up briefly, are as follows:

A) Take salt water baths in your tub.

B) Improve circulation and muscle tone with hot foot baths.

C) If you're not too far from the sea, go ocean bathing in mild weather.

D) Remember that bathing in the cool waters of upland lakes and streams is invigorating, too.

E) Take sun baths of limited duration until you have acquired a protective tan.

F) Take sun-and-air baths in your own home from fall until spring.

G) Bathe in the nude to restore the normal function of the skin, and for the psychological feeling of liberation and freedom there is in being unclothed. If you must wear something, put on as little as possible.

I recall the anecdote about a visit Sir Winston Churchill made to President Roosevelt at the White House. Knowing that Churchill invariably slept late, FDR waited until nearly noon before knocking on his distinguished guest's door.

"Come in," Sir Winston cheerily called.

As the President opened the door, he was suddenly taken aback with astonishment at the sight he saw. There sat Churchill in a comfortable armchair, contentedly smoking a cigar, and wearing not even a fig leaf!

"Didn't I tell you," Sir Winston nonchalantly remarked, "that we English have nothing to hide from you Americans?"

Activities and Exercises as Rejuvenators, Restoratives and Invigorators

7 While exercise will not extend your life span, it will invigorate and rejuvenate you, and keep you looking, feeling, and acting young, well beyond middle age.

Why does exercise provide these benefits? Because it sends the blood circulating through muscles and joints. It activates the brain by providing it with more oxygen. It improves digestive and bowel action, calms the nervous system, and alleviates circulatory ailments.

Exercise is one of the three essentials for keeping the body in top-notch condition. The other two are eating and sleeping. All three must be practiced every day for the most satisfactory results. You rarely pass a day without eating and sleeping; but, if you are an average American, you often let days go by without any real exercise. This imbalance in your health program is definitely unfavorable. Your body needs exercise, just as it needs rest and nutrition, day in and day out.

don't force yourself

Exercise must never be attempted when you are physically tired, or when you have not had sufficient rest. It should always leave you refreshed and raring to go. Don't feel that exercise must wear you out to do you any good.

Doc Silvers says: "For maximum benefit, exercise should be a pleasure, not a chore."

the right way to breathe

You would think that *homo sapiens*, that fine, upstanding, intelligent creature who, with his mate, reign as king and queen of the animal world, would know how to breathe. After all, they have been practicing it for several million years. Nevertheless, 90% of us don't breathe properly, thereby suffering from a lack of oxygen, and all of the ills attendant thereto.

If you want to really feel like a new man—or a new woman—the first thing you should do is learn to breathe. It is not at all difficult, I assure you. And once you get on to it, you will feel more vibrantly alive than you ever did before. What's more, you'll keep on feeling that way.

belly breathing

Some people believe that when they exercise they should start out with the most strenuous program on the books. Then, when they find it too much effort, they give it up as an excessive strain on their physical capabilities. The more sensible plan is to begin with the easiest exercises, gradually adding more difficult workouts as you go along.

The simplest exercise of all, and one of the best, is belly breathing. Diaphragmatic or belly breathing can be learned easily by anyone. It is a purposeful exercise, and should not be confused with normal or automatic breathing, which goes on even when we are unconscious.

Most of us have been taught the wrong way to breathe since early childhood. This unnatural expansion of the chest, when we inhale deeply, restricts the physiological, aspiratory action of the rib cage. When correctly done, the diaphragm performs the aspiratory or suction action connected with breathing.

Forget that you have a chest, or if you can't do that, imagine that it is paralyzed. Lie supine on your back, legs flexed and extended, and stretch every muscle taut, then relax it: first the right leg, then the left; right arm and left arm. When each limb has been relaxed, try to separate your head from your body by neck stretching, without any movement of the rest of the body. Stretch hard, toes toward the foot of the bed, and head toward the headboard. Then relax. Each of these stretches should last a full minute, or until you feel the muscles tiring. You are now ready for your belly breathing.

Home Rx:

1) Place right hand on your belly to measure its proper action as you breathe.

2) Inhale through both nose and mouth, slowly and deeply, gradually inflating the belly, as indicated by the upward movement of your hand.

3) When you feel that your human bellows is fully inflated, without any undue effort or strain, relax completely and allow the belly to deflate automatically.

4) Lie limp during this elastic rebound of the body wall, diaphragm and lungs.

5) After complete deflation, when your hand has lowered as far as possible without any muscular effort, draw in another breath the same way.

6) Repeat this breathing exercise from six to a dozen times. It will stimulate you in the morning and tranquilize you at night.

what belly breathing does for you

For an example of proper breathing, watch an infant in its crib. You will see its abdomen going up and down with each complete ventilating cycle. Another example of the belly breather can be found in the singer, actor, or public speaker. Each of these performers has learned the advantages of abdominal control in the projection of the voice, in addition to its circulatory benefits.

The diaphragm is a muscle which normally operates automatically. However, this elastic partition, separating the upper (thorax) from the lower (abdominal) body cavities, is also to some extent under the control of your will. Every time the diaphragm contracts it reduces pressure in the chest cavity, and increases it in the abdominal cavity. The lowered pressure in the chest causes air to be sucked in, and stimulates the flow of blood to the heart from the large veins in the neck, arms, abdomen and legs. Each contraction of the diaphragm presses down upon the stomach, liver, gall bladder, spleen, intestine, and the vast network of veins surrounding them. Only by breathing naturally, from the belly, can you avoid the stagnation of a large portion of the total volume of your blood. Belly breathing pumps some of the blood from the abdominal area, upward toward the heart, at each breath. Proper blood flow like this helps prevent many of the common complaints developed by chest breathers, such as bile stoppage in the liver, varicose veins in the legs, and hemorrhoids.

Belly breathing is helpful to the stammerer and stutterer, assisting him to control his speech. It is beneficial to those past middle age suffering from high blood pressure, who would like help in lowering it. And it is an aid to the insomniac as a safe substitute for sleeping pills.

Doc Silvers says: "The belly has a number of uses, from the digestive to the decorative, but one of its chief functions—as a breathing apparatus—is too often forgotten."

you can swim your way to better health

There are many light sports which provide non-strenuous exercise, among them archery, badminton, boating, croquet, horse shoe pitching, hiking, medicine ball, and tennis doubles. Each is good in its way, one developing arm muscles, another leg muscles, others agility and coordination. However, swimming is the best all-around exercise, as it develops all the muscles, and can be done without strain because of the water's support.

Most of us do a little swimming at the beach in summer, and

let it go at that. Like any other exercise, swimming should be done consistently, outdoors in good weather, and indoors during the cold season. The swimmer should learn not to fight the water, but allow it to buoy him up and help propel him along. He should always inhale through the mouth and exhale through both nose and mouth. When tired, change to an easier stroke, or turn over and float. It is foolish to get over-tired or chilled, and excessive sunburn can, of course, be dangerous.

exercise after your shower

If you don't patronize a pool, but do all your bathing at home under the shower, you can still give yourself a little workout. After the shower, bend forward and try to touch the bottom of the tub with your fingertips, without bending the knees. (Make sure to have a safety mat under your feet to prevent slipping.) Do a dozen bends each time, reaching further and further each day, until eventually you are able to touch the mat.

Next, remaining in the bent forward position, place hands on knees and press the knees alternately inward and outward, as though you were cutting a figure eight on ice skates. This is a good exercise to promote more balanced posture, and to relieve back pain. Repeat a dozen times.

The human body is normally in perfect balance, and proper exercise should keep it so. The litheness of the ballet dancer or acrobat comes with years of daily practice. We cannot all be as agile as they are, but we can try to become as balanced and limber as our muscular structure will permit.

Doc Silvers says: "The more you do for your muscles, the more they will do for you."

Liven up While Lying Down

If you'd like to take a quiescent approach to exercise, there is no need even to get out of bed, for you can liven up while lying down. There are any number of exercises that can be performed while lying down. They can be done in bed on a firm mattress or one with a bed board, on an army cot stretched with canvas or nylon, or on a rug spread with a blanket. Here are four exercises that will give you a good five-minute workout.

Flat on Your Back:

KNEE FLEXING

1) Raise the right knee back toward the chin as far as possible, almost touching the chest.

2) Lift right leg upward, with toes turned down like a ballet dancer, then slowly drop it to the mattress.

3) Repeat with left leg.

4) Alternate left and right ten times.

This is an excellent relief for chronic backache that will not respond to any other form of manipulation or exercise. Naturally, it cannot cure a diseased condition; but it can relieve muscle spasm or stiffness, or lack of coordination in muscular pull.

SHOULDER CURLING

1) Tuck hands under small of back, palms down.

2) Tighten abdominal muscles and lift the head, to get a better view of your toes, pulling shoulders and elbows off mattress.

3) Count to four.

4) Return to starting position.

5) Repeat five times.

BICYCLE RIDING

1) Rest shoulders and head on mattress, arms at sides.

2) Raise legs and hips high above the head.

3) Balance body on shoulders, neck and back of head.

4) Place hands under hips, with elbows braced against mattress.

5) Pump legs vigorously, as though pushing bicycle pedals, while counting up to ten.

6) Return to starting position.

7) Repeat ten times, taking an imaginary ride down the Atlantic City boardwalk.

HIP TWISTING

1) Keep legs straight and together, arms stretched sideward at shoulder level.

2) Lift left leg at right angles to body.

3) Allow leg to fall across body to right and try to put the toes in the right hand, the way a baby would.

4) Raise left leg up straight once more.

5) Return to starting position.

6) Repeat same movements with right leg, keeping body and other leg straight, and shoulders flat.

It is not wise to attempt all the exercises the first day for the maximum number of times. To avoid muscle strain and exhaustion, do them twice the first day, four times the second, and so on, up to five, ten, or a dozen, or whatever the stipulated number.

Don't attempt this entire series of lying down exercises the first day, either. Preferably, do the "Flat on Your Back" series the first week, adding the "Sit-up Set-ups" the second week, the "Belly Whoppers" series the third week, and the "Sideways" series the fourth week. When you have them all down pat, the entire stint should be accomplished in just 15 minutes.

After that, if you feel like it, you can add some exercises done standing up, at the side of the bed.

Sit-up Set-ups:

STRETCH OVER

1) Sit up with legs spread, hands resting on knees.

2) Bend over at waist, extending arms down legs toward toes as far as possible.

3) Count to three.

4) Return to starting position.

5) Repeat ten times.

SIT-UP

1) Lie flat on back, feet slightly apart, arms at sides.

2) Sit up to vertical position without lifting feet. Pretend there is a weight holding them in place.

3) Return to original position.

4) Repeat five times.

EXTENDED SIT-UP

1) Lie on back, legs together, arms extended above head.

2) Bring arms forward over head, rolling up to sitting position, pulling on an invisible rope.

3) Put hands on legs and slide them forward to ankles.

4) Count to three.

5) Return in same manner to starting position.

6) Repeat five times.

ELBOW STRETCH

1) Sit up with legs spread, fingers clasped behind neck.

2) Bend forward from waist, bringing elbows as close to mattress as possible.

3) Count to three.

4) Return to original position.

5) Repeat 12 times.

Shortness of Breath:

If you note shortness of breath following vigorous exercise, don't be alarmed. It is normal, and the medical term for it is "tachypnea." If your breathing and heart beat are not back to normal within five to ten minutes after exercising, then you should check with your doctor. Your discomfort may be due to simple body flabbiness, malnutrition, or obesity. In fact, the latter is often the culprit, since you are doing your daily stint with an extra load equal to the amount of your overweight. Shortness of breath may also be caused by altitude, air pollution, or improper ventilation of the room.

Doc Silvers says: "Exercise combined with proper diet can reduce excess poundage. Then, should you decide to become a weight lifter, the weight you lift won't be your own."

BACK ARCH

1) Lie face downward, hands beneath thighs.
2) Lift head, shoulders and legs, like a fish out of water.
3) Return to original position.
4) Repeat ten times.

ELBOW PUSH

1) Lie face down, legs straight, shoulders raised by resting weight on forearms, hands clasped.
2) Lift body by raising it parallel to bed, resting weight on elbows, forearms, and toes.
3) Lower body to original position.
4) Repeat five times.

KNEE PUSH

1) Lie face down, legs together, knees bent so that feet are raised, upper arms close to body, bent forward at elbows, hands palms downward.
2) Push body off floor, with weight on hands and knees, until arms are fully extended and upper body is on a straight incline of 90 degrees, like the centerpiece of a sundial.
3) Count to three.
4) Return to original position.

LEG LIFT

1) Lie face down, legs together, extended straight.
2) Lift head and right leg.
3) Lower to original position.
4) Lift head and left leg.
5) Lower to original position.
6) Repeat ten times, alternating right and left legs, as if skin diving.

how to make a progress report

By the time you have reached this point in your exercise program, you should be able to perform your daily calisthenics with a minimum of exertion, and less shortness of breath and rapidity of pulse. You will feel the beneficial results in your daily activities. One of the functions of exercise is to put you in such good shape that your ordinary bodily requirements no longer tire you. There'll be a smoother line to stomach and hips, more zest in your actions, and a sparkle in your eyes.

Doc Silvers says: "The best two-way stretch is not the one ladies buy at the lingerie counter, but the one you get from your daily calisthenics."

Sideways for a Change

THE SCISSORS

1) Lie on right side, right arm extended above head, and head resting on it.

2) Raise left leg stiffly about two feet, then lower it.

3) Repeat five times, like a snipping scissors.

4) Turn over on left side, left arm extended above head, head resting on it.

5) Raise right leg about two feet, then lower it.

6) Repeat scissor action five times.

ELEVATED SCISSORS

1) With right side turned toward floor, support weight on extended right arm and hand, and the side of right foot, using left hand to keep balance.

2) Lift left leg until it is parallel with mattress.

3) Lower leg to starting position.

4) Repeat five times.

5) Turn to left side and repeat five times with right leg.

THE RIGHT ANGLE

1) Lie with right side of body turned downward, right arm and leg extended, head resting on arm.

2) Lift left leg up at right angles with right leg (or as close to right angles as possible without undue strain).

3) Return to original position.

4) Repeat six times rapidly.

5) Turn to left side and repeat seven times with right leg.

Resistance Exercises

This form of exercise, called "isometrics," consisting of pressure and weight resistance, originated in hospitals and rehabilitation centers. Some are known as gravity-eliminated exercises. The arm is suspended in a sling, and the patient exercises it with a pulley mechanism; as the muscles grow stronger, weights are added to the pulley apparatus. The patient sits while doing this exercise, so that the rest of the body doesn't need to move.

When these isometric exercises were introduced to the general public a few years ago, they were found to have great appeal because they didn't involve a lot of jumping around. They look easy, and they are. Remember, though, that they are just muscle developers. They do not give you all the circulatory and other advantages that you obtain from the more active calisthenics, such as the other type of resistance exercise known as "isotonics." Isotonics is a modification of isometrics, which allows a wider range of movement for each part of the body, and maintains or increases the extent of joint motion, while also strengthening the muscles involved. Chinning yourself on a horizontal bar is an example of this type of exercise.

Let's assume you've done your exercises on the bed, and have just got up; but you don't feel equal to chinning yourself. Remove the pillowslip from your pillow, and you are ready to begin your isometrics.

A

1) Place pillowslip around back of neck, pulling ends forward with the hands.

2) Push neck back hard against slip, while pulling ends forward firmly, counting up to six.

B

1) Make a sling of the pillowslip, and step into it with the right foot.

2) Press against slip with ball of foot, while pulling upward with hands.

3) Count up to four, then repeat with opposite foot.

C

1) Pass pillowslip around the small of the back, and pull ends forward with hands.

2) Tighten abdominal and back muscles to resist forward pull of hands.

3) Count to six, then relax.

Now discard the pillowslip and lie down on the floor, face downward, arms at sides, legs extending under the bed.

D

1) Lie face down, arms at sides, palms up.

2) With hips kept flat to floor, lift right leg, knee straight, and push heel hard against frame of bed.

3) Count to three.

4) Repeat with left leg.

enjoy yourself more by being fit

Many people would prefer to get all their exercise by dancing, bowling, coasting, or playing picnic games. This kind of activity is fine, but it must be supplementary to the basic daily exercise which is done faithfully to keep you in trim. Such daily calisthenics, even when done lying down, is no particular fun, I'll agree. The fun you derive from it comes when you go dancing, bowling, coasting, or relay racing, and find that you can enjoy yourself more because your muscles are in shape. You can play better, tire less easily, and have the fun of being a doer, rather than a spectator.

Doc Silvers says: "Take one hour of exercise and recreation for every eight hours of work, and you'll face the next day with enthusiasm and pep."

Putting More Spice in Your Life by Putting More Variety in Your Diet

8 You don't have to be a nutritionist to figure how to get your daily vitamin requirements from the foods you consume. Here is what you need each day to obtain the basic vitamins, to which you add a variety of other foods to make up the total calories your particular constitution requires.

BASIC DAILY DIETARY

Milk	1 pint
Egg	1 medium
Meat, fish or fowl	3 oz. without bone
Potato	1 medium
Green, leafy or yellow vegetables	½ cup
Other vegetables	½ cup
Citrus fruits	1 serving
Other fruits	1 serving
Bread, white enriched or whole wheat	3 slices
Cereal, whole grain or enriched	⅔ cup cooked or 1 doz. dry
Butter or margarine	1 tablespoon
Total:	approx. 1,300 calories

With this fundamental diet, you can't go wrong unless the balance of your daily caloric consumption consists largely of one type of food, such as starches or sweets, both of which we consume far too much. "Variety's the very spice of life," as William Cowper said, and it particularly applies to food.

natural foods to make you feel better

Several natural foods should be included in your daily diet, and your own taste will decide how you prefer them. The richest natural food source of the B Complex, especially thiamin or B1, is wheat germ from plain wheat as it comes from the thresher. The best source of riboflavin or B2 is milk and its derivatives: skimmed, buttermilk, evaporated, yogurt, and cheese. Don't use cottage cheese as it cheats you of vitamins A and D, which are removed in making cream. You can fortify your cereal with lecithin and brewer's yeast, one tablespoon of each. The yeast, besides being a high-quality protein, has many of the B vitamins, and is also a good source of iron and phosphorus. Lecithin is an essential part of all animal and vegetable cells. It is obtained from soya beans, which have been defatted, as a bland, granular powder soluble in water and milk. It has been used for ages as part of the soya bean diet of the peoples of the Far East. Soya bean has substituted for milk, being commonly known as "oriental milk," and is fed to babies who are allergic to cow's milk. Lecithin is one of the most important constituents of the soya bean. It is responsible for dissolving the fatty deposits in the blood vessels, hence preventing and reserving the atherosclerotic process previously described. Research workers have only recently shown that soya bean lecithin is capable of preventing clots from forming in the blood vessels. In conjunction with the use of estrogen, mentioned earlier, it has been possible to markedly reduce the incidence of coronary artery disease and cerebral vascular disease. Thus we have moved forward still another step in the prevention and treatment of vascular degenerative diseases, which are presently the greatest killers in western civilization. By supplementing your diet with wheat germ, brewer's yeast, and lecithin (all obtainable at natural food stores), you have the richest supply of vitamin B Complex, and the best food prevention of blood vessel disease.

how to avoid insecticides

The problem of insecticides is becoming more troublesome every year. Our fruits and vegetables are sprayed with harmful chemicals which defy the common cleansing process of ordinary washing with running water. Often when you are otherwise in good health, you suddenly have a spell of diarrhea for which you cannot account. If you recollect what you ate the day before, you may note that it included a tossed green salad which you enjoyed. One of the many causes of gastrointestinal upset, it occurred because the greens had been sprinkled with an insecticide, which irritated your intestinal tract much like a whopping dose of castor oil.

The only properly effective way, which I have advocated for years, to clean fruit and vegetables and thoroughly remove the offending pesticide is by the following technique:

Home Rx:

1 oz. (two tablespoons) of dilute hydrochloric acid added to 1 quart of cold water. (Ask your druggist for 1 pint of 10% diluted HCL.)

Immerse all fruits and vegetables eaten raw in the solution for 30 minutes; then rinse thoroughly under the cold-water faucet. Since our stomachs contain at least 2% HCL, no bad effects can result from this cleansing method. The diluted acid dissolves the metallic salts that were previously sprayed on the food by the farmer in his zeal to keep the food for you and not for the meally worms.

why the staff of life can be lifeless

So it is with everything we get from storage today. Flour is devitalized by removing all the essential vitamins and minerals, so that the bugs will not get at it, since even the bugs have more sense than to waste their time eating paperhanger's paste. That's all flour is when you remove the wheat germ, the bran, and the part called middlings, which is fed to hogs and cattle. Yes, it retards spoilage and keeps the bread "fresh" for a longer time; but the bugs wouldn't touch it with a ten-foot pole—and neither should humans. The situation is a bit better today since, by law, the baker puts back a few of the most essential vitamins. He calls it "enriched" bread, and the younger generation—who have never had the pleasure of tasting good home-made bread fresh from the oven—think it means that the baker has added extra food values to a natural product, whereas, if the truth be known, he takes out a whale of a lot more than he puts back in.

Since bread is a common staple consumed daily by most people, it behooves us to make certain that we get it in the form which Nature intended: complete with natural wheat germ, bran, vitamins B1 and E, and all the others essential for our well-being. In buying bread, it is wise to forget the whites altogether, even though they are the so-called "enriched," and make your selection from the variety of tasty dark breads, such as whole wheat, rye, pumpernickel, bran.

The skin of the potato is the richest portion of the "Irish fruit." Baked potato, therefore, is better for you than boiled or mashed. Likewise, the most beneficial part of citrus fruits is right next to the skin where the bioflavonoids (vitamin P) abound. Throw away this portion of the fruit and your doctor will have to prescribe the missing vitamin. Your druggist will then dispense to you for a fee the very same substance that you nonchalantly tossed into the garbage. While the peel is bitter, it can be sweetened and candied, or purchased in that form, and tastes delicious.

raw vs. cooked food as a health measure

All animal and plant life have always existed on Nature's raw food. Only *homo sapiens*—which means "wise man," a terminology we often don't live up to—has learned to kindle a fire and cook his food. The vegetarian animals, like the hoofed horse, cow, antelope, reindeer, elephant, rhinoceros, hippopotamus, and so on, all thrive on raw grass and grain.

We know from experimental proof that raw food contains many

important factors which are destroyed by heat. For example, milk as it comes from the animal's breast is richer in enzymes and vitamins than heated milk. At least three factors present in raw milk are destroyed by pasteurization: an arthritis-prevention factor, an ulcer-prevention factor, and an anemia-prevention factor. If you were to compare animals fed on raw milk with those fed on heated milk to the third and fourth generation, you would find that the former were much healthier than the latter, with bone and muscle structure showing greater strength and durability. That mysterious and powerful *vis a tergo* (force that pushes) which drives all living creatures, is much more pronounced in animals on diets of raw rather than heated milk. In this very connection, prospective mothers should remember that the formula food which many babies are fed from birth **does not contain many of the beneficial factors found in breast milk.** Despite the advances made, infant mortality in the U.S. is still appreciably higher than in other civilized countries; and one of the important contributing factors is that today most American women do not give their babies mother's milk.

Doc Silvers says: "**Mothers, to give your child the best opportunity for a long and healthful life, forget formulas, and nurse it at your breast as Nature intended.**"

Since raw milk is much better, then why do all civilized countries heat-treat milk for human consumption? Simply because it is the lesser of two evils. Since it is difficult to guarantee the cleanliness and wholesomeness of raw milk, it must be pasteurized. Just as we destroy many important factors in other protein-rich foods by heating, so we must sacrifice these health-giving enzymes and vitamins to protect us from germ and parasitic infestation. In the present economic status of the world, it is highly impractical to indulge everyone with the blessings of ideal food consumption.

Modern improvements in the storage of food, with particular emphasis on refrigeration, have appreciably increased the safety factor of the most easily spoiled foods, the proteins. The use of irradiation in small amounts has helped to eradicate the infestation of the trichina spiralis (parasitic worms) from pork and ham. The carcass of the recently slaughtered animal is hung up, and power-ful rays from an X-ray machine are directed at it for just a few seconds. While the rays do not destroy the female worm, they render its ovaries incapable of ovulation. Thus instead of a thousand offspring for each ingested trichina, only the original female remains alive; and since it cannot multiply in our intestines, it does no harm.

As a double safety factor against a possibly diseased animal, it is most important to cook pork thoroughly in order to destroy any live parasites. Today, as a further safeguard, most countries require the boiling of all garbage fed to hogs. This simple precaution has cut down the transmission of disease in Germany, where raw blutwurst and liverwurst are common delicacies.

So we must cook animal flesh, even though several important beneficial factors are sacrificed thereby. It is better to be protected against disease in this way rather than keep on taking chances daily of seriously impairing our health.

know when to eat

In ancient Rome, people really ate only once a day, instead of three times, as we customarily do. For breakfast, the Roman had a glass of water, and nothing else. At noon, he lunched on a small piece of meat and a little fruit. In the evening, to make up for this sparse diet, he banqueted and stuffed himself until he was ready to burst. Lying on a couch, with his head toward the table, he gorged on food and wine for hours on end. When he was full, he often tickled his throat with a feather so that he could induce emesis and start all over. And when he was finally finished, to express his appreciation to the host, he burped loudly. No wonder that, in 476, the empire fell to the Goths, for the Romans were undoubtedly too fat and full to fight.

Today we customarily have three meals daily. Doctors, nutri-tionists, and dieticians are pretty generally agreed that breakfast should be substantial, followed by a light lunch, with the main meal in the evening. While I have no quarrel with that regimen,

I believe that it can be improved upon in several ways which will help your digestion, sharpen your appetite, make you actively inclined, and better your general health. In addition, you can thereby control your weight more easily.

1) Eat when you are hungry. It is Nature's signal that she wants you to stoke the furnace and, as you know, you can depend on Nature.

2) I advocate eating more often than three times a day, a half-dozen meals, if you wish.

3) Eat less at each sitting, which you will naturally do when you eat more frequently.

4) Don't ever eat until you are stuffed, as the Romans did at their banquets. If you are over 35, it can kill you because of the extra work it puts on your heart.

5) At home, serve smaller portions of the main entrée. Three ounces of edible meat (not counting bone, fat, and gristle) is the size portion recommended by all nutritionists.

6) When a guest at someone else's home, request a small serving of meat. If you are given too much, don't be hesitant about leaving some on your plate; and you needn't make apologies for it, either.

7) When dining at a restaurant, forget the full-course dinners and order from the à la carte menu. It doesn't cost as much and, more important, you'll eat less if you refrain from ordering everything from soup to nuts.

8) Select restaurants with care. The basic slogan of the restaurant trade is "good food and plenty of it," and many restaurants pridefully advertise their giant cocktails and large portions of food. A doctor friend, who is particularly interested in diet because many of his patients are rich and fat—two characteristics which often go together—told me of recently dining at one of New York's finest and oldest restaurants. For the entrée, he ordered sauerbraten which, according to the menu, consisted of prime eye of round that had been marinated in wine for 30 days. He was served five thick slices, totaling at least a pound of solid meat, with lots of gravy, potatoes, and a vegetable. He estimated that this main course

ran to over 2,000 calories; and though he is a hearty eater, he was forced to leave three slices of meat. This piling up of food on the groaning board is both wasteful and shameful, particularly when one reflects that well over half the world's population exists on a starvation diet. So don't eat at restaurants which serve gargantuan courses that you can't finish—though you must pay for them—without suffering from gastritis, or even getting a heart attack. Instead, patronize places distinguished for good food, served in sensible portions, in pleasant surroundings, at reasonable prices. Not only will you avoid waste, save money, and keep healthier, but you'll live longer, too.

Doc Silvers says: "To wine and dine is fine as long as it doesn't turn pleasure into pain."

learn to use natural laxatives

Constipation is a far too common disturbance of the digestive tract amongst Americans. Millions take laxative pills every day. The average American is "pill happy," and the statistics prove it. In the past decade, consumer expenditures for drugs and drug sundries have more than doubled. A decade ago, we spent under $2 billion, while today it's over $4 billion. In the same period, the expenditure for consumer advertising of drugs and remedies has tripled. Laxatives are a substantial item in these figures.

Laxatives are irritating, afford only temporary relief, and are habit-forming. If you are the victim of a "lazy colon"—or *think* you are, which amounts to the same thing—I have a brief bit of advice for you which will make you healthier, happier, and save you a tidy sum besides: Don't take anything for constipation unless you are so advised by a doctor. Chances are a hundred to one that, if you observe the simple basic rules of nutrition and diet, you will have no need for laxatives. *All* food has a stimulating effect on the stomach and intestines and, in more or less degree, is laxative in physiological action. The coarser the food, the more irritating to the mucosa of the intestinal tract, thus the more laxative it becomes. Only the blandest of food, like boiled rice and raw peeled apple is permitted in the acute stage of diarrhea. The pectin in raw apple is what your doctor would prescribe for you in medicinal doses for this distressing condition.

The less residue left after digestion is accounted for by the fact that certain foods, like cheese and the white of eggs, are the least laxative of all. Most people believe that milk tends to constipation. However, this assumption has no basis in fact whatever. Known to nutritionists and dieticians as "the nearly perfect food," milk is actually neither laxative nor binding in its action. There is only one element which keeps milk from being the "ideal food," and that is iron. However, this lack is easily remedied. Babies thrive on milk alone, and can continue on it exclusively provided the vitamins destroyed by heating are replaced, and iron is added from other food sources.

Any restriction in food intake naturally causes a letdown in bowel function. It is the quantity of food, as well as the variety, which makes the bowel function more or less active. Foods which contain such indigestible residue as fiber, bran, and cellulose, as in skins, seeds, coarse vegetables and fruits, leave a bulkier residue and that, of course, acts as a more vigorous stimulant to the bowel.

Doc Silvers says: "**Unless directed by your doctor to refrain from some particular food that may not agree with you due to allergy or disease, you can eat any food without fear of a bowel disturbance as long as it is appetizing and wholesomely prepared.**"

Roughage is, as a rule, the bête noire (black beast) of older people. As they head toward their sixties, the large bowel gets small pockets or diverticulae, which harbor undigested material. In this condition, coarse, indigestible food can cause trouble. However, it is not a disease; it is part of the aging process. Only when the weakened walls of the bowel fill with fecal matter and inflammation ensues do we call it diverticulitis. A ruptured diverticulum acts just like a ruptured appendix symptomized by an acute abdominal pain.

Otherwise, it matters but little how you prefer your food. It may be baked, boiled, broiled, fried, roasted, stewed, either well done, rare, or raw (without parasites). Just the fact that you eat with enjoyment adds greatly to the digestibility of your food. In a later chapter, where insomnia is discussed, you will learn that sleeplessness is principally caused by worrying about it. In the very same way, mere anxiety over the state of one's bowels, and about timing and promptness, is enough in itself to produce constipation.

don't be a worry wart

The most common factor of constipation is the bad habit of worrying over the action of the bowels. The regular peristalsis (contractions) are waves which knead and mix the food and propel the mass through the digestive tract. Dogs will, in strange surroundings or in slightly uncomfortable situations, show a cessation of peristalsis that may last for two or three hours. Similar effects have been observed in humans. Any kind of anxiety, worry, fear, anger, irritation, annoyance, or other unpleasant emotion is enough to upset, delay, or stop the normal process of digestion, spoil the appetite, and inhibit or retard normal peristalsis. Even insignificant anxiety, such as comes from disturbing telephone calls, catching a train, the fear of being late for appointments, the difficulty of avoiding encounters with people one doesn't wish to see, all tend to slow down the whole alimentary function. A clear conscience and a jovial disposition are the best aids to digestion, and the only really satisfying bowel regulators. They require no prescription, and cost not a penny.

don't be a slave to laxatives

Perhaps you recollect the delightful quip that goes like this:

> John: Only a fool can be certain of anything.
> Harry: Are you sure?
> John: Positively!

Nevertheless, I am as certain as I can be that, if you are a victim of the laxative habit, you can cure yourself of it promptly without any trouble whatever. It will take only a couple of days, and cost just a few cents. First, swear off laxatives immediately. Not tomorrow—today! Then use this simple, inexpensive prescription:

Home Rx:
1 tablespoon of malt soup extract
Take up to three times a day, as needed for normal regularity, mixing it in milk, soup, or any fruit drink. In addition, drink two glasses of buttermilk daily.

The malt soup extract is obtainable at drug and health food stores. Use it for several days, not more than a week, and you will find that your normal bowel regularity will continue of itself without any special medication of any kind. The malt soup extract is the mildest form of laxative, adding something to the bowels which prevents putrefaction, and advantageously changing the flora of the lower digestive tract. The extract and the buttermilk are all that are needed to give normal laxation, even to those who are most constipated. From then on, you will have no further trouble.

Doc Silvers says: "Food is fuel that feeds the furnace, which then eliminates the waste. Stoke it daily with the nutrients that Nature has provided in abundance, and it will need little or no overhauling and repair."

How to Lose Weight Without Losing Vigor

9

There is only one way to reduce successfully and safely. It is medically approved, and it works every time. Furthermore, if you continue to observe a proper dietary, you needn't worry about ever getting fat again. There are just two basic rules:

reduce gradually!

The fallacy in crash diets is that they expect fast results which are humanly impossible of accomplishment. After all, if it took you ten years to put on ten pounds of excess fat, how can you hope to get rid of it in ten days? Since, as has been shown, overweight is a serious malady, let's be sensible about it and reduce gradually over a reasonable period of time. To insure that your efforts are crowned with success, make this reasonable goal your aim:

reduce one pound a week!

If you put on ten excess pounds in ten years, you can expect to regain your normal weight in ten weeks; if you put on 20 pounds in 20 years, you should get back to your proper weight in 20 weeks, and so on. Using a little elementary arithmetic, this means that, by basing your weight reduction program on this reasonable regimen, *you will be reducing 50 times faster than you added the poundage!* So forget the crash diets, which never work out in the

103

long run, and start on a reducing program that makes good sense.

Still doubtful that you can do it? Then perhaps the relations of a classic case will encourage you. The Scotsman George Cheyn was born in 1671. When he reached 30 years of age, he had attained the stupendous weight of 448 pounds. By gradually reducing his daily intake of food, he eventually lost nearly 300 pounds of fat. And by remaining on a sensible diet, he lived into his eighth decade, and kept well until the end.

This extraordinary experience is as amazing as anything ever reported by Ripley. While the life expectancy at birth nearly three centuries ago is unknown, it is a certainty that it couldn't have been much over 30 years, as indicated by these later figures, which have been recorded:

LIFE EXPECTANCY AT BIRTH IN THE UNITED STATES

Year	Male	Female
1850	38.3	40.5
1900	48.23	51.08
1960	67.4	74.1

Note that in a little over a century, man's life expectancy at birth has increased 29 years, while woman's has increased 34 years.

If George Cheyn, 300 years ago, without the benefit of modern drugs, with little or no sanitation, and without the vast accumulation of knowledge in medicine, nutrition, and dietetics that has been amassed since then, could shed 300 pounds and live to a ripe old age, certainly you can get rid of your comparatively few pounds of excess weight as gradually, sensibly, and surely as he did.

Doc Silvers says: "To paraphrase an old song: 'Every little bit subtracted from what you weigh, makes just a little bit less.'"

know your desirable weight

Before you can start on an effective reducing program, you must know what has been found to be your most healthful weight, considering your height and frame. A glance at the accompanying weight table will give you this figure. Take a 3 x 5 index card or a small sheet of paper and write your desirable weight at the top. A good way to keep this record is to paste it with a piece of scotch tape on the inside of your medicine cabinet door. Weigh yourself in indoor clothing on the bathroom scales, and make a note of the date and your present weight. Then weigh yourself once a week, not more often, and record it.

how to determine your daily calorie allowance

Now that you know what you should weigh, you must find out what your daily caloric consumption should be for your age and weight. Reference to the calorie chart will give you that amount. While counting calories can be deadly dull, don't be too concerned about it as you will be given ways to circumvent that daily chore. Though when you are at your desirable weight you will want to keep your food consumption within your calorie allowance, you can easily develop simple habit patterns—which we will go into shortly—that will make it unnecessary for you to count calories day in and day out.

CALORIE ALLOWANCES FOR INDIVIDUALS
OF VARIOUS BODY WEIGHTS

Men

Desirable weight in pounds	Calorie Allowances		
	25 years	45 years	65 years
110	2500	2350	1950
121	2700	2550	2150
132	2850	2700	2250
143	3000	2800	2350
154	3200	3000	2550
165	3400	3200	2700
176	3550	3350	2800
187	3700	3500	2900

NEW WEIGHT TABLES

Weight in Pounds According to Frame (In Indoor Clothing)

	HEIGHT (with shoes on) 1-inch heels Feet Inches		SMALL FRAME	MEDIUM FRAME	LARGE FRAME
	5	2	112–120	118–129	126–141
	5	3	115–123	121–133	129–144
	5	4	118–126	124–136	132–148
DESIRABLE	5	5	121–129	127–139	135–152
WEIGHTS	5	6	124–133	130–143	138–156
FOR MEN	5	7	128–137	134–147	142–161
of ages 25	5	8	132–141	138–152	147–166
and over	5	9	136–145	142–156	151–170
	5	10	140–150	146–160	155–174
	5	11	144–154	150–165	159–179
	6	0	148–158	154–170	164–184
	6	1	152–162	158–175	168–189
	6	2	156–167	162–180	173–194
	6	3	160–171	167–185	178–199
	6	4	164–175	172–190	182–204

	HEIGHT (with shoes on) 2-inch heels Feet Inches		SMALL FRAME	MEDIUM FRAME	LARGE FRAME
	4	10	92– 98	96–107	104–119
	4	11	94–101	98–110	106–122
	5	0	96–104	101–113	109–125
	5	1	99–107	104–116	112–128
DESIRABLE	5	2	102–110	107–119	115–131
WEIGHTS	5	3	105–113	110–122	118–134
FOR WOMEN	5	4	108–116	113–126	121–138
of ages 25	5	5	111–119	116–130	125–142
and over	5	6	114–123	120–135	129–146
	5	7	118–127	124–139	133–150
	5	8	122–131	128–143	137–154
	5	9	126–135	132–147	141–158
	5	10	130–140	136–151	145–163
	5	11	134–144	140–155	149–168
	6	0	138–148	144–159	153–173

Women

Desirable weight in pounds	Calorie Allowances		
	25 years	45 years	65 years
88	1750	1650	1400
99	1900	1800	1500
110	2050	1950	1600
121	2200	2050	1750
128	2300	2200	1800
132	2350	2200	1850
143	2500	2350	2000
154	2600	2450	2050
165	2750	2600	2150

how to reduce without starving

Now don't get scared; Doc Silvers isn't going to hurt you. The several methods of weight reduction we propose are not going to deprive you of essential foods. And you needn't go around with "a lean and hungry look," as Cassius did in Shakespeare's *Julius Caesar*.

You can lose a pound a week by reducing your daily food consumption by just 500 calories, amounting in a week to 3,500 calories, which equal one pound of body fat. And in doing it, you can still get your full amount of proteins, and all of the essential vitamins and minerals.

Check your calorie allowance on the chart, and deduct 500; that will be your daily nutriment until you have reduced to your desirable weight, as indicated on the weight table. For the purposes of illustration, we will take average figures. The average man has a daily allowance of 3,000 calories; the average woman has 2,200 calories. Most crash diets call for a food intake of only 900 calories daily. This is impossible, nonsensical, and dangerous. But any person with an ounce of determination can consume 500 calories less a day without any trouble whatever, if the suggestions given below are followed.

The *Basic Daily Dietary* previously given totals only 1,300 calories, *and* it includes meat, egg, milk, butter or margarine. You stick to this foundation diet, even while reducing, to insure that you are getting all the food essentials every day. Now in the case of an average man, he will reduce his calorie allowance from 3,000 to 2,500 calories, leaving him 1,200 additional calories above the basic dietary. An average woman will reduce her daily allowance from 2,200 calories to 1,700, leaving her 400 extra calories to consume above the basic diet. It is evident, therefore, that both of them have enough additional calories to play around with so they need have no fear of becoming as emaciated as the cigarette fiends in circus sideshows.

recognize these protein protectors

This weight-reducing program also insures that you obtain your daily requirement of protein. Of Greek derivation, it means "of first importance." Every animal, including man, must have an adequate supply of protein in order to grow and maintain itself. As proteins are the principal constituents of the active tissues of the body, which are dependent upon food protein for these indispensable substances, the quality and quantity in the diet are of prime importance. The daily protein requirement for men is 70 grams; for women about 60 grams. Use the protein table as a guide in selecting your meals so that you make certain of getting the amount of protein you need each and every day. In this connection, note that protein is pretty tricky stuff, and you should consume the proper human requirement, not more or less, as any deviation from the norm can get you into trouble.

PROTEIN IN COMMON FOODS

Food	Serving	Grams of Protein
MILK OR EQUIVALENT		
Milk, whole or skim	1 cup	9
Cottage cheese	2 oz.	10
Cheddar cheese	2 oz.	12
Ice cream	3½ oz. container	2

MEAT, FISH, POULTRY, EGGS

Fish	3 oz.	24
Beef	3 oz.	20
Liver	3 oz.	19
Fowl	3 oz.	20
Tuna fish	3 oz.	25
Egg	1	6

VEGETABLES AND FRUITS

Lima beans	1 cup	16
Peas	1 cup	20
Greens	1 cup	4

BREADS AND CEREAL

Bread, white or dark	2 slices	4
Macaroni or spaghetti	1 cup	6
Cooked cereal	1 cup	5

use this prudent diet

Consider this—if you reduce your daily calorie intake by 500 calories a day, you can lose a pound a week. That is very little, so I am not going to belabor you about it as I am sure you can do it. For example, if you dropped from your diet a chocolate drink and a cup of baked custard, you would reduce your daily consumption by approximately 500 calories right there. Or you might pass up a hamburger and a piece of gingerbread, which also amount to about 500 calories. Refer to a calorie chart, select a few items totaling around 500 calories, and omit them from your normal calorie allowance.

If you find that you are not losing a pound a week, I can point without hesitation to where the trouble lies: you are consuming too large portions of the main dish. The recommended serving of meat, poultry and fish is three ounces, without bone, gristle or visible fat. I realize that this nutritional directive is going to create consternation among a lot of he-men, but that is enough for any man, no matter how much hair he has on his chest. And if he doesn't observe this fundamental dietary rule, he is going to stay a fatty for the rest of his life, which will be short as he is certain to succumb before his time to a heart or circulatory condition, or one of the other drastic diseases to which the overweight are prone.

There are several fine restaurants in Manhattan that list sirloin steak twice on their menus. One item is described as "under a pound," the other as "over a pound." Now a broiled sirloin steak, which is all solid meat, weighing around one pound, is more than enough for four people! When a man consumes a steak of that size at one sitting, he is literally digging his grave with his teeth. Four ounces of tender steak taste as delicious as 16 ounces, just as a small container of ice cream is every bit as tasty and sweet as a whole quart. So why emulate Henry VIII and be a glutton?

Doc Silvers says: **"Be prudent, eat what is sufficient for good health, and you will enjoy a long and contented life, meanwhile avoiding many of the ills of mankind."**

vary your menus

Modern American women are good cooks. I wouldn't say that their mothers and grandmothers were more proficient in the kitchen. In fact, what with all the good food available, electric refrigeration, and other modern appliances, it could well be that today's housewife is a better cook than her mother was. "If this be treason, make the most of it." What's more, today's homemaker is not chained to stove and washtub as her female forebears were. Science has liberated her from kitchen and basement, and it's all to the good. Now she can prepare a savory meal—and I am not speaking of frozen TV dinners, which are a horror!—in an hour or so, instead of taking all day.

Nowadays the housewife can take advantage of a greater variety of foods than ever before. And by varying the diet, quantity becomes of less importance. Put the emphasis on quality, taste, and variety, and you will find that you enjoy your food more while eating less. Let us look briefly at the values in basic foods which usually constitute the main entrée.

Meat, fish and eggs are rich in essential protein, iron, and B complex, in addition to calories. Eat fish or shellfish more frequently; not just on Fridays, but several times a week. Fish is distinct in taste, one from the other; and it is appreciably cheaper than meat. Some like it for breakfast as well as lunch or dinner. The people of the British Isles, being surrounded by sea, go for kippers at breakfast, and fish and chips (fried potatoes) any time of the day or night. While you are reducing until you get down to your proper weight, increase your fish dishes. It will help you to knock off that extra fat as fish, pound for pound, contains about half the calories of beef. In addition, fish is an excellent source of polyunsaturated fatty acids, and also provides the daily supply of iodine. To guide you in the selection of fish while you are on a reducing program, and afterwards, too, here are the percentages of fat and the caloric content of common varieties:

COMPOSITION OF FISH

Fish	Percent of Fat	Approx. Calories per 3 oz. Serving
Bass	2%	90
Bonito	7%	140
Cod	Trace	60
Flounder	1%	65
Haddock	Trace	60
Herring	13%	125
Mackerel	12%	165
Pike	1%	75
Salmon	17%	120
Shad	10%	150
Trout	2%	85
White fish	7%	140

COMPOSITION OF SHELLFISH

Clams	1%	75
Crabs	3%	80
Lobsters	2%	80
Mussels	2%	85
Oysters	2%	75
Scallops	Trace	65
Shrimps	1%	75

All fish oils are highly polyunsaturated. This is today interpreted by medical science to account for the relative absence of vascular diseases amongst the fish-consuming races. The Oriental and the Eskimo consume large quantities of polyunsaturated fats in the form of fish oils, and have been found to be comparatively free of coronary artery disease.

Poultry is richest in polyunsaturates, and should be eaten frequently, whether on a reducing diet or not.

Veal, like poultry and fish, is low in fat, and should be alternated with them for variety as they each have a distinct flavor of their own.

While reducing and, for that matter, even when you are maintaining your desirable weight, beef, pork and lamb, all high in saturated fats, should be curtailed to not more than three meals a week.

Organ or variety meats, such as liver, heart, and kidney, are excellent sources of essential vitamins, and should be eaten more frequently when not contraindicated.

Avoid the fatter meats, such as pork, bacon, sausage, corned beef, and pastrami. Serve only the leaner cuts of meat, and always trim off the visible fat. Most important of all, remember, is to keep portions to three ounces, as recommended by all nutritionists and dieticians.

As for eggs, one a day is indicated for all who are not cholesterol conscious. Interestingly enough, in this connection, eggs that contain twice the amount of polyunsaturates as in regular eggs have already been placed on the market. A special vegetable feed formula has evenly balanced the polyunsaturates with the saturate fats.

Doc Silvers says: "Vary your menus from day to day, taking full advantage of the wealth of good foods available from all over the country and the world. By so doing, you will eat less and enjoy your meals more, thus enabling you to maintain your desirable weight without struggling to reduce year in and year out."

why your biggest enemy is your sweet tooth

You can substantially lower your daily calorie consumption by reducing your intake of the carbohydrates, which include starches and sugar. If you avoid them assiduously, you can easily reduce your food consumption 500 calories daily by this method alone. Sweets are the big bugaboo; the largest tooth we Americans have is our sweet tooth which, unfortunately, modern dentistry has not yet discovered how to extract. The quantity of sugar (including sweets and the sweetening in processed foods) recommended by nutritionists and dieticians for adults is ten ounces a week. However, we consume three times that amount, and the figure continues to rise. In 1910, the annual per capita consumption of sugar was 75 pounds; today it is 100 pounds. That is equivalent to about 50 pounds of body fat. Therefore, if you cut your consumption of sugars and sweets in half, you would still be getting more than your nutritional need, and you'd eliminate 25 pounds of excess body fat in a year just by making your sweet tooth behave.

avoid bread and butter and lose 28 pounds

The staff of life spread with butter or margarine is a standard food in the daily diet. According to the basic dietary, the recommended consumption of this staple is three slices of bread and a tablespoon of butter or margarine each day. These total 280 calories and, in a year, reach the staggering total of over 100,000 calories. Translated into body fat, it is 28 pounds, so if you eat no bread and butter or margarine, you can reduce your weight by that amount.

summarizing your pound-a-week program

In order to lose one pound in weight each week, you must reduce your nutritional allowance by 500 calories a day. A number of practical and simple methods have been given to accomplish this reasonable and sensible goal, as follows:

1) Serve the recommended portions of meat, fowl, and fish, namely three ounces without bone, gristle, or visible fat.
2) Trim off all visible fat before cooking.
3) Use vegetable oils in cooking and for salads.
4) Favor lean meats and fish.
5) Serve fish more frequently.
6) Have organ or variety meats upon occasion.
7) Go easy on starches.
8) Cut the consumption of sugar and sweets in half.
9) Do without bread and butter until proper weight is reached.
10) Drink coffee or tea without cream or sugar.
11) Don't eat sweets at the coffee breaks.
12) And here is one more for good measure: Don't eat snacks until your weight reduction program has been completed.

By following these suggestions, selecting those which are easiest for your mental and emotional makeup, you will have no difficulty in reducing a pound a week until you are at your desirable weight. Besides, because of the nature of these methods, you don't have to count calories constantly since you are bound to reduce gradually, safely and surely until you have attained your goal. You will refer to a calorie chart principally to look up the calorie content of various foods in order to select those which are low in calories, carbohydrates, and fat. Only if you find that you are not losing weight steadily, will you need to keep track of your calorie consumption for a short while to locate where the fault lies. Once you are generally familiar with the nutrients in common foods, knowing which to prefer and what to avoid, you won't need to refer to a calorie chart again.

how advances in food processing can keep you thinner

The future in foods is now beginning to appear at our supermarkets. Your favorite foods are camouflaged to taste as well without fat as they did with the natural fat content. Peanuts are freed of their unsaturated fats so that you can eat more of them and still remain trim. A handful of these protein-rich peanuts, which register 84 calories before removal of the oil, now contain only 17 calories, and are just as tempting. Thus you are able to indulge your appetite, and still hold down that avoirdupois.

For America's weight-watchers, these low-calorie foods, in ample supply, will soon eliminate the present preponderance of failure in weight reduction. Then there'll be no more temporary tries at a crash diet, with the usual return to the old regimen after a few weeks of denial and sacrifice.

The new low-calorie foods take into consideration the need for flavorful and easily digested nutrients, which are so often missing in the fad foods. They are made to have body as well as bulk in order to satisfy your hunger pains with a minimum of calorie content. Vegetables and herbs replace the flavor of the fats removed. Special taste chemists are constantly at work trying to replace the flavor which was present in meats and poultry before subjection to 2,000 degrees of infrared lamp heat in processing. The flavorful herbs and vegetables, such as mace, oregano, ginger, pimentos, peppers, Italian tomatoes, onions, garlic, which are all low in calorie content, are added to render the converted food more palatable. The noncaloric sweeteners enable you to enjoy natural fruits in preserved form. You can avoid over 50% of high-calorie sugar in the general run of preserves now on the market.

Dr. Frederick Stare, Chairman of the Department of Nutrition at the Harvard School of Public Health, has stated that, "The newer low-calorie foods, tasty and appetizing, provide pleasure in dieting, even to the texture of the food when one is chewing. They can be just as nutritious as regular foods. You can lose with them if you remember that, in losing weight, the number of calories you take in is all that counts in the long run."

This is excellent advice. Now that practically every food in the dietary is produced in low fat and/or low-calorie form, and most stores stock them, little effort is needed to reduce your daily food requirement by 500 calories until you reach your best weight, and to keep at that desirable weight thereafter. The suggestions made in this chapter do not comprise a fad diet since you follow physiological precepts. And you can be certain of a trim waistline simply by favoring low-calorie foods. This prudent diet completely eliminates the crash and "on again off again" reducing regimens.

Homo sapiens is an omnivorous animal by nature, and must mix his foods thoroughly to obtain all the necessary factors for health and longevity. So beware of any special dietary which requires a limited form of food intake, and does not permit the broad variety of foods that are necessary and good for you. While it is true that the crow lives primarily on stolen eggs from the nests of smaller birds, it also eats whole grain and worms. Next to the parrot, the crow is one of the longest lived of all birds. In captivity, the parrot lives primarily on sunflower seeds as a snack between meals. For health and longevity, he also requires a mixed feed which will supply him with all the vitamins, minerals and protein that his body requires daily. The parrot has been known to live over a century, but to do so he must have a varied and most nutritious diet— besides a very good master or mistress.

The pantry of the future will be so different from the food we are accustomed to that we will not recognize the many new items on the shelves of our supermarkets. The present emphasis is on the polyunsaturated fats. The food industry has taken serious cognizance of the increasing desire to reduce hard or saturated fats, and simultaneously raise the liquid or polyunsaturated fats in our dietary. Already on the market are special butter substitutes that are nearly as free of saturated fats as the vegetable oils, though slight hydrogenation is still necessary to give them the consistency of butter.

We can now get milk products practically free of saturated butter fat. Skimmed milk is being used to make a preparation of acidophilus milk which is of advantage to those who need to reduce the putrefactive bacteria in the colon. By adding lactose or milk sugar, honey or malt extract, molasses or fruit sugar, to your intake of acidophilus culture or yogurt, you help grow the beneficial antiputrefactive organisms in the colon. Much relief from gas and bloating may thus be obtained.

Ice cream can now be made from safflower seed oil, and so contains mostly polyunsaturates. Manufacturers of hard shortenings have added polyunsaturated oils to counteract the process of hydrogenation. The dairy and meat industries are probing into the future diets of an enlightened populace, and there will be many changes made in our food supply in the years just ahead. Pigs are omnivorous like humans, as has been said, and enjoy eating a most varied diet. Polyunsaturated oils added to the porker's diet will produce meat which is less saturated. If the cost is not prohibitive, pork can be produced which is far more polyunsaturated. Unfortunately, this is not so easily accomplished in the ruminants with multiple stomachs, like the cow and sheep, as a chemical process in the second part of the stomach pouch converts the polyunsaturated into saturated fat. Special feeding and breeding can, however, do much to breed cattle that are more muscular than fat. At present, animals are fattened up just before slaughtering. Elimination of this fattening up process would cut down on the saturated fat content of meat. This will require changes in our meat grading system. The "prime" or tastiest meat is fattest, followed by "choice," which is less fat, and finally, by "commercial," which is least fat. Since the lean meats are more stringy and less tender, a new process has been devised to tenderize the carcass by injecting enzymes which break down the tougher muscle and fibrous tissues.

The dairy industry has a more difficult problem ahead of it. While the fat can be removed from milk in skimming and cheese production, it has the butter, which is rich in saturated fat, on its hands. Increased sales in cottage cheese, farmer cheese, and pot cheese already show future trends. Butter is rapidly being replaced by margarines that are high in polyunsaturates. It is not a simple matter to change the saturation of butter by feeding the cow different nutrients. And it is impossible to change chemically, once it is churned. However, the dairy industry is facing this contretemps with courage and imagination, and it is certain to make definite progress in the years to come

dietary of the future

One thing is now positive about our future diets. We can reduce the amount of cholesterol in the blood stream by eating more poly-unsaturates. The commercial trend, therefore, will be towards the production of food which is least saturated in fat content. Provided that the taste of this new dietary is attractive, it will replace our present-day diet, and so cut down on the diseases of the heart and blood vessels. You will be able to eat as much as you like, and yet keep your weight within normal bounds. While it sounds like Utopia, it is all scientifically a problem of the daily consumption of calories. A low-calorie diet will permit you to eat more freely of foods which otherwise would be either restricted or taboo. So we can now look forward with high hopes to the dietary of the future. It is certain to do much to prevent presently prevalent strokes and heart attacks, and thus help to prolong a healthful life. Meanwhile, follow the suggestions given in this chapter regarding a prudent diet, and you will more fully enjoy all the years of a longer lifetime.

Doc Silvers says: "A small, tender steak of choice or prime quality is more tasty and enjoyable than a large, tough steak of commercial grade. The gourmand eats to fill his stomach, while the gourmet eats to satisfy his appetite and get the utmost pleasure out of good, well-prepared meals."

How to Relax Without Drugs

10 The foundation stone of "the good life" is regularity in all things: eating, working, resting, exercising, and relaxation. Unfortunately, many do not so organize their days as to get the most out of them in accomplishment, satisfaction, and enjoyment. Far too often we hear people complain that they haven't time for reading, for a round of golf or some other healthful recreation, or time to relax. Men and women who are successful in their work, frequently conduct their private lives in a most disorderly fashion.

Doc Silvers says: **"If businesses were as poorly organized as some lives, there would be a lot more bankruptcies."**

The purpose of this book is to indicate how you can be healthier, happier, and enjoy a long, active life to the end of your days. One of the essentials is relaxation integrated into your regular daily schedule. Don't say that you haven't time to relax; take time by the forelock and *make* time for relaxation. In this busy, productive, prosperous nation, time has become the master of man. We wouldn't accomplish as much, and we wouldn't be quite so rich, but we would be happier and live longer if we adopted the ancient oriental philosophy: "Time is your servant." It is not difficult to put into effect; simply plan your days ahead, and observe the program as dutifully as you do the obligations of your vocation.

Doc Silvers says: **"Man's responsibilities are multifold: to his work, to society, to God, to his family, and not the least of these is his responsibility to himself."**

learn to relax

Any habit is formed by doing the same thing over and over again. And it is just as easy to form a good habit as a bad one. In fact, it should be easier since a good habit is beneficial while a bad habit is destructive. One of the most rewarding of good habits is relaxation. As a matter of fact, the person who knows how to relax *gets more work done in less time* because he approaches his job with greater enthusiasm and zest.

get up with the birds

The fundamental habits which should all be regularized are: ingestion, elimination, work, exercise, relaxation, and rest. The sleep habit pattern has two determinants: the hours of rest you require, and the time you have to get up in the morning. If you arise at seven o'clock, and need eight hours of sleep, it is obvious that you should retire at eleven in the evening; and if you maintain that schedule until it has become an ingrained habit, you will.

Ben Franklin's familiar couplet: "Early to bed and early to rise, makes a man healthy, wealthy, and wise," has long been a schoolbook maxim. I have observed an interesting example of this among my patients and friends who are bird watchers. They are not all wealthy, to be sure, but they are intelligent, in good health, observant, and considerate of their fellow creatures, whether they be birds or human beings. So if your sleep pattern is irregular, try getting up with the birds, and you'll have no trouble falling into a deep and untroubled sleep at a reasonable hour each night. You won't need a nerve-jangling alarm clock to awaken you, either. Instead, you'll automatically get up on time, rested and refreshed, with your eyes wide open and your mind alerted to the work and play of the day ahead.

Your eating habits should observe a definite pattern, too. As was said in discussing foods earlier, the time to eat is when you are hungry and, once your other basic habits are regulated, you will have a good appetite when you draw your chair up to the table. The important factor is to be completely relaxed before the meal. Upon occasion, having had a hard day, or perhaps a spat with your spouse, you are all keyed up and tense. In that case, use this sure-fire relaxer.

Home Rx:

A hot drink a half-hour before a meal.

Have whatever drink you prefer, but it must be hot. Prune juice, taken hot before a meal, serves a double function. First, the heat relaxes you; secondly, it acts as a mild laxative if you are inclined to be constipated. A cup of bouillon is relaxing, too. A teaspoon of plain gelatin, without flavoring or added sugar, may be mixed into the cup of bouillon, thus supplying a high concentration of protein rich in most of the amino acids.

A heated drink does more to relax you than a tranquilizer in any form. Have a cup of hot soup, if you prefer. The primary role of hot drinks is their relaxing effect. Even coffee and tea, though containing the psychic stimulant caffeine, are antispasmodic and, therefore, relaxing when taken before a meal. The hot drink has several functions. It stimulates the gastric juices, while a cold drink retards them. It dilates the vessels lining the stomach and intestines, and so enhances the process of absorption. It satisfies your hunger more readily than cold drinks because of the relaxing effect. In health, the temperature of the body is always the same. When you put something cold into your stomach, it must first be brought up to the body temperature of 98.6 degrees, thus requiring the expenditure of energy, and so temporarily interfering with normal body processes. When you are healthy, this extra expense of energy is not discernible. However, should you have a little trouble in emptying the gall bladder, a characteristic pain over the upper right side of the abdomen may ensue. Therefore, if you suspect difficulty with any of your digestive organs, forego cold drinks.

hot vs. cold drinks

In this connection, it is interesting to note what happened in England when our soldiers arrived during World War II. Hot tea has long been the favorite drink of the British; and gall bladder trouble was uncommon in England then. However, the Americans brought along their penchant for ice-cold drinks, and many of the English cultivated the habit. Pronto, an increase was observed in gastro-intestinal upsets, with a specific involvement of the gall bladder. Spasm of the sphincter muscle, which controls the exit of the bile from the gall bladder, resulted. Thus one of the basic principles in physical medicine and physiology was confirmed: Heat relaxes muscle fibers, while cold causes them to contract.

Cold drinks retard the chemical reactions which must take place in the stomach and intestine. Iced drinks not only further delay the enzymatic reactions necessary to good digestion, but may also overstimulate the musculature, so that the sphincter muscles at the outlet of the stomach, and those that control the passage of the bile from the liver may contract. It is then that you will note heartburn, indigestion, and even pain in the region of the gall bladder. Iced alcoholic drinks are particularly likely to produce these physical phenomena.

Americans like their beer good and cold. And now, to make matters worse, it has become fashionable to order scotch, bourbon "on the rocks." Other nations don't have the fetish for cold alcoholic beverages that we do. A friend who recently covered the pubs in London—"purely in the interests of research," so he claims —told me that the beer and ale on tap were too warm for his taste; even when he ordered cold bottled beer, it was fetched from a tank of water in which the ice had long since melted, and was still not frigid enough to suit him. The fact of the matter is that iced beer and liquor won't cool you off; instead, they are bound to heat you up because of their alcoholic content.

Doc Silvers says: "A cold drink is refreshing, especially in warm weather. But the best thing to cool you off and relax you is a flavorful hot drink at any time of the year."

quick cure for indigestion

Should you suffer from simple indigestion, due to overeating or eating while under tension, you can easily get immediate relief with this simple remedy.

Home Rx:
  3 drops Essence of Peppermint
  Mix in ½ glass of hot water
Sip slowly and you will experience a relieved feeling of warmth, and your discomfort will soon be forgotten. Medicinally, this drink is known as a carminative or stomach tranquilizer, which quickly relieves the bloated, gassy feeling that makes one so uncomfortable after a big meal. Its primary action is to stimulate the emptying time of the stomach, and so relieve any irritation due to swelling and congestion. The reaction of the stomach mucosa combined with the peppermint essence is also beneficial as an antispasmodic. Remember that heat will relax your muscles, whether or not they are controlled by your own volition. Once food or drink enters the esophagus on its way to the stomach, you no longer have any control over it. Everything that happens from there on is entirely managed by the involuntary nervous system. Excessive activity of the secretory glands can mean too much hydrochloric acid in the stomach. It is this excess acidity which may lead to the discomfort of heartburn or, carried further, it can be the causative factor in ulcer formation and slowness in healing. That is the reason for taking alkaline mixtures for neutralizing the excess acid in stomach and duodenal ulcers. Here the advice of your physician must be followed to make certain that you are dieting properly, and not overdoing the neutralization of the normal stomach acid.

Doc Silvers says: "The processes of the constitution are governed by various checks and balances so that the body, like a ship, can sail on an even keel through both calm and stormy weather."

an easy way to avoid nausea

That queasy feeling in the stomach, accompanied by an impulse to vomit, is occasioned in many ways, of which seasickness (mal de mer) is the most familiar. You can become nauseated during any form of transit: bus, subway, car, ship or plane. One can even feel like "up-chucking" because of homesickness (mal du pays). The impelling desire to throw up also results from overeating. This sickly feeling, however promoted, can often be aborted, and the vomiting avoided, by a simple, relaxing massage.

Home Rx:

As soon as you feel nausea coming on, stroke downward from the back of the ears, with the fingers of your hands, to the upper part of the neck, and along the sides of each jaw. Either do it yourself or, even better, have a companion perform this gentle, relaxing massage for a minute or two, and the sensation of nausea will be immediately alleviated.

how to relieve peptic indigestion

Peptic indigestion differs from simple indigestion, which was discussed a moment ago, in that the former results from an insufficiency of acid in the stomach secretions. Fortunately, it can be readily relieved with this simple hot drink.

Home Rx:

2 teaspoons of vinegar (preferably apple cider)
1 tablespoon of honey
Mix into a glass of hot water and drink slowly

You will find this a pleasant drink that relaxes you as all hot drinks do, thus aiding your digestion and enhancing your feeling of well-being. The vinegar insures the essential acidity needed to augment the enzymatic action of the stomach pepsin. In addition, the honey contributes to the general relaxing effect. Today doctors are advising the increased use of honey for better muscular tone, which includes the improved function of the heart muscle, an important factor, what with the prevalence of cardiovascular diseases.

a three-way cocktail

Should you be low in iodine as a dietary supplement, which you well may be unless you eat seafood regularly, you can add two drops of an aqueous solution of 5% elemental iodine and 10% potassium iodide (ask your pharmacist for Lugol's solution) to this hot drink. Thus with a simple, nonalcoholic cocktail, you profit three ways: you relax, you obtain your daily requirement of iodine, and you relieve any peptic indigestion besides. A Manhattan or Martini can't give you any of these benefits, while this health-giving cocktail provides dollars in health value for only a few cents.

Doc Silvers says: "One of the amazing things about physical medicine is that simple, inexpensive home remedies not only relax your body, but your heart and mind as well."

Relaxation, as was said earlier, should be integrated into your regular daily schedule. The trouble with us fast-moving Americans is that, while we program our important activities, we don't plan our relaxations, which are of equal consequence in maintaining physical and mental health. Here then are some suggestions which, if followed, will help to smooth out your busy days, avoid flare-ups and frustrations, keep your life on an even keel, and make days on end much more enjoyable.

20 PROVEN WAYS TO RELAX, BE HAPPIER, AND LIVE LONGER

A Daily Program

1) Don't rush in the morning. Instead, get up fifteen minutes earlier so that you can prepare for the day in a more leisurely manner.

2) Don't read the morning paper during breakfast as it may disturb your digestion and upset you emotionally. Instead, have a pleasant conversation with other members of your family.

3) Don't run to catch a bus or subway; there will be another along in a few minutes. This is a must for those over 35. It should also be observed by younger people as it establishes a healthful habit for the later years.

4) Schedule your day so that you are consistently on time for work, appointments, and dates. You will be respected and appreciated for your promptness, and it also saves wear and tear on your heart.

5) If you have a strong difference of opinion with someone about a phase of your work, don't argue it out face-to-face. Instead, turn to something else, and later, when you have calmed down, present your case fairly and straightforwardly in a memorandum.

6) Keep your work tools in a neat, orderly fashion so that, instead of frequently getting into a tizzy, you can find what you want when you want it. That goes for those in business and for housewives, too.

7) At coffee breaks, and at other times as well, favor hot drinks, even in warm weather, for their relaxing effect. If you are a homemaker, remember that you should have regular coffee breaks, too.

8) If possible, have your business lunch with a pleasant companion. Follow this principle for all meals and, if it can be avoided, don't eat alone. Agreeable conversation at the table slows down the consumption of food, assists the digestive process, and makes meals more enjoyable.

9) Allow a few minutes after lunch for a stroll around the block.

10) Arrange your work schedule so that you do quieter tasks for the hour following the lunch period, thus helping your digestion. A good idea is to plan your next day's duties at that time.

11) Proceed with your duties at the same steady pace throughout the day and you will get more done than if you work in fits and starts. Besides, you will avoid emotional stress, and thus protect your heart.

12) Don't watch the clock and rush through your work at the end of the day. Do things right, avoid mistakes and accidents, and stay a while after quitting time, if need be. It won't kill you while rushing eventually may; and if you plan your work properly, frequent overtime shouldn't be required.

13) Homemakers should space out their heavier chores. For example, don't spend all day in housecleaning. Instead, clean mornings only, and engage in lighter activities afternoons. In this way, your daily expenditure of energy will be more evenly distributed, and you will avoid overexhaustion thereby. It is upsetting, to say the least, for a tired husband to be greeted by a tired wife at the end of the day.

14) When you come home from business, take a freshing shower or tub, followed by a relaxing hot drink. Then take a short stroll with your dog before dinner.

15) Have a good dinner with your family, and then relax for a half-hour or so. An excellent idea is to keep some light literature—paperback books are inexpensive—beside your favorite chair: mysteries, adventure, romance, or humor, as you prefer. When you want to relax for a few minutes, read several pages.

16) Don't spend all evening staring at the television tube. Plan one hour of recreation, preferably an outdoor activity. Then watch your favorite TV show.

17) Have a midevening snack, if you wish, but don't go over your daily caloric requirement. Have crackers and warm milk, cookies with tea or coffee, anything that isn't too rich and sweet.

18) If you don't have an evening snack, have a hot drink before bedtime.

19) Remember to kiss your spouse good night.

20) Go to bed, forget the cares of the day, and enjoy a restful night's sleep.

How to Get to Sleep
Fast and Rest Easier

11 I have, in my practice, met many insomniacs, and, believe me, they are a sight to behold. Let me introduce you to a typical case.

He tosses and frets through the night, worrying at the prospect of getting up in the morning, completely exhausted, and unable to face the rigors of a new day. He begins to fear that constant lack of sleep will inevitably bring on mental as well as physical afflictions. His resistance being lowered from insufficient rest, he becomes a ready victim to various infectious diseases. Increasing nervous insomnia shatters his nerves, and he expects that it will eventually lead to complete mental disintegration.

By this time, he is well on his way to becoming a hypochondriac, fancying himself a sufferer of various imaginary ills. He begins to have alarming pains, here, there, and everywhere. He rushes to a drugstore and pleads with the pharmacist to give him something to put him to sleep. He tries the sleeping potions advertised on radio and television. All to no avail.

Now he's got the heebie-jeebies. He notices that his extremities get cold at night, not realizing that it is the normal result of lowered circulation while at rest. His hands get clammy and his feet perspire. He is positive that he is on the verge of complete physical and mental collapse.

Does this graphic picture of a typical insomniac shock you? I wouldn't be surprised if it did. However, you needn't be too sympathetic toward him because of his dilemma. The fact of the matter is that the all-too-common belief that protracted insomnia leads directly to physical and mental ruin just doesn't hold water. Many mature patients have said to me in all sincerity that they haven't slept through a single night for 20, 30, or even 40 years. However, I invariably find that, despite their conviction that they haven't slept for decades—some having been without sleep through both world wars!—it has apparently done them no physical harm. These good folk who, to put it politely, are simply deluding themselves, are like the "pleasingly plump" women who, when I suggest dieting, declare with vehemence: "Why, doctor, I hardly eat a thing!"

you don't need sleep!

That's right. What you need is rest! Sleep will do you little good if you fight it all night long. What actually tires you is not the lack of sleep, but your emotional distress over your inability to "pound your ear" on a soft pillow. If you fail to sleep, and are constantly fagged out, it is not from wakefulness, but rather from worrying about it. If you really make up your mind to it, you can rest as well without sleep as with it. But you must keep your body quiet and your mind calm. Under normal conditions, you don't necessarily require eight hours of sleep. What you need is eight hours of rest in bed.

The rhythm pattern you have developed in early childhood determines how much sleep you should have for the maximum benefit to your particular constitution. So don't concern yourself with how many hours you sleep. Instead, concentrate on how much rest you get. If you take that attitude, you will never become an insomniac.

should you take sleeping pills?

Prescribing sleeping pills to induce sleep is indicated *only* when there is a need to get essential rest in case of a major illness. To conserve the energy the body must have to fight an infection, a hypnotic or sleeping pill may help toward a more rapid recovery. But for the normally healthy individual who, like some of my patients, "hasn't slept for years," it is folly to take a sleeping pill. What's more, it is extremely dangerous since narcotics are so insidious in their effect that the victim is entrapped before he knows it.

In the early stages of the drug habit there is a feeling of well being. The brain is pleasantly sedated, and all worries are forgotten for the time being. However, small doses soon fail to satisfy, and have to be increased, raising the cost from $25 to $50 a day!

At first, the victim attempts to fight against the habit, but the struggle is ineffectual. Then steady mental and physical deterioration sets in. The addict becomes intensely self-centered, and subordinates everything to the satisfaction of his uncontrollable desire for the narcotic. He becomes untrustworthy, immoral, and depraved. His intelligence is reduced, and his memory is faulty. Finally, he becomes the lowest of the low, having no interest in life outside of his addiction. His desire is so great that he will do *anything* to get the money for drugs—he will even murder. The Police Department of the City of New York says that the vast majority of burglaries and robberies are committed by drug addicts.

Burn these four proven facts into your brain, and you will always be on guard against becoming a victim of sleeping pills and other deadly dangerous narcotics:

1) Introduction to a drug is usually accidental.
2) The drug habit is very quickly acquired.
3) Only ten percent are permanently cured of drug addiction.
4) *All* sleeping pills can become habit-forming.

Proof that most insomniacs are just kidding themselves is shown by the fact that the prescribing of a simple sugar pill (placebo), having no effective drugs whatever, is enough to cure most cases of insomnia, no matter how long-standing. But even the innocent, harmless sugar pill can be habit-forming, if it produces the desired result. *Anything* that gives us the feeling of well being and elation known as "euphoria" is capable of inducing a habit formation.

how to tell a habit from an addiction

It is important to distinguish between habit and addiction. A habit may be good or bad. Rising at a regular hour each day is good; consuming too many sweets is bad. Addiction, on the other hand, is *never* good.

When, for example, you break a bad habit like smoking, there is no fear of becoming physically ill. Mentally, you suffer from the deprivation until you become adjusted to the change in habit pattern. And you may increase in weight by substituting food for smoke, as many do. But you won't get out-and-out sick, as you would with a narcotic addiction.

The reason you enjoy a cigarette is primarily physical. The nicotine on inhalation, on contact with the mucous membrane, is absorbed into the blood stream. When it reaches the liver, it liberates the stored sugar (glycogen). It is this physiological response to the drug which accounts for the mental and physical lift following a smoke. Fortunately, this habit may be broken without physical harm.

An addiction to narcotics or alcohol, however, cannot be cut off simply and easily. The cellular structure becomes so attached to the habitual use of the drug that sudden stoppage may very well mean disaster to the constitution. Scientifically, we must gradually reduce the dosage of the medication in small measured amounts, meanwhile carefully noting the organic reaction of the patient. For instance, to prevent delirium tremens in the chronic alcoholic, it is extremely important, after a long spree, to taper off the patient gradually.

I am reminded, in this connection, of a case during the era of prohibition, when I was young in practice and experience, as well as in years. An "old soak" went off on a "lost weekend" every now and then on bootleg liquor. While on one of these binges, the manager of the hotel where he was staying called me in to straighten him out. One glance at the patient told me that he was on the verge of delirium tremens and beginning to see pink elephants. A whopping dose of a hypnotic drug (paraldehyde) served to quiet him down, and he was able to get a good night's sleep.

The next morning, however, he began to shake again, and was threatening to go into convulsions. I knew what his suffering body craved, and wrote a prescription which permitted a druggist to dispense one pint of whiskey. I then placed the patient under the care of a registered nurse, and instructed her to give him one tablespoon of whiskey every four hours. It took three days of gradually reduced intake of alcohol to keep this unfortunate man's body and soul together. This typical case demonstrates the difference between a *habit* and an *addiction*. Alcoholism is the result of an addiction, while cigarette smoking, on the other hand, is a habit.

This episode had an amusing epilogue, though it didn't seem so to me at the time. A week or so later, I received a telephone call from the alcoholic's wife. Under the circumstances, I couldn't blame the poor woman for being upset. But when she irately took me to task for having prescribed whiskey, no less, for a confirmed alcoholic, I was flabbergasted. I tried to explain that "a nip of the snake that bit you" is sound medical therapy; but to no avail, and she threatened to sue. Finally, I suggested that she check with her family doctor. He corroborated the scientific aspect of my treatment, and thus a lawsuit was avoided.

When you take any drug to induce sleep, you invite a habit formation. However, taken in moderation, not every night, and for essential purposes, a hypnotic can be a valuable aid in tiding you over an illness. It may be indicated before and after an operation for the rest and relaxation it provides in time of crisis. But *never* take a drug except under the advice of a physician, who knows when it is the lesser of two evils. If you take it because modern life is so strenuous that you feel you cannot stand the strain, you are inviting trouble—and possibly disaster. When you are tempted to take a pill, be guided by the ancient Greek proverb: "Sleep is the only medicine that gives ease." So forget drugs, and learn to sleep by natural means.

how to get easier sleep and more rest

The best way to fall asleep is to do it completely unconsciously. Don't get all upset and say to yourself: "Oh, my God, I'm going to lay awake all night again!" If you stop caring whether you are falling asleep or not, you will soon find that you are in the arms of Morpheus before you know it. Never consciously search for sleep, as it is very fickle, and will fly away if you pursue it. Just lie quietly in bed, and firmly put away the discomforts of the day. Concentrate on the pleasant things that have happened, and consider how much more fortunate you are, whatever your circumstances, than millions of others.

The sensible thing to do is to take for granted that the body knows by instinct how much rest it requires. As soon as you accept the fact that loss of sleep is of no physical consequence, you will no longer be an insomniac. Since the cause of insomnia is primarily psychic, the only logical cure is to substitute a new frame of mind which accepts sleep for what it is, and no more.

Napoleon, who had defeats as well as victories, declared that he always slept soundly. He kept, he explained, different ideas in various drawers of his mind. "If I wish to sleep," he said, "I shut up all the drawers, and I am asleep." Napoleon was right—it's as simple as that.

"But," you may protest, "I'm no Napoleon," and I won't argue with you. But if you think you have troubles, you should have had his. And you are emulating his military tactics when you fight off sleep, which is exactly what confirmed insomniacs do.

Think back to your childhood. When you were a youngster, I am certain that you had no difficulty falling into a deep sleep the minute your head hit the pillow. Insomnia is extremely rare in the early years. Being physically tired from the day's activities brought on the need for rest. An accumulation of the products of fatigue, which is a chemical reaction, resulted in that tired, sleepy feeling which came over you naturally. You stretched your arms, yawned, and it was all you could do to keep your eyes open. When you were four years old, you had no trouble sleeping a dozen hours a night. In your teens, you slept nine to ten hours daily. As an adult, about eight hours is considered the normal and desirable duration of bed rest, though it is not a hard-and-fast rule.

There are several tried-and-true methods to induce sleep. You may require one, two, or all of them to obtain the blessed slumber you need. Select those which apply to your particular makeup, and experiment with them. After all, if you have been an insomniac for years, it is well worth the attempt for the chances are ten to one in your favor that you can quickly overcome sleeplessness once and for all.

hot drinks make sleepy people

A hot drink is the best of all nightcaps. Coffee and tea are stimulants, both containing caffeine. But there are lots of people who can drink them before bedtime, and still get a good night's sleep. Whether or not you can have them at night depends upon your mental gymnastics. It goes like this:

a) If you believe that coffee or tea keeps you awake, it will.

b) If you think that they don't keep you awake, they won't.

If you are among the former, but crave the coffee flavor, use one of the caffeine-free substitutes which are readily available. But for a really relaxing drink, mix a tablespoon of honey and a teaspoon of lemon juice in a glass of boiled, piping hot water. It tastes good, it is good, and it does you good.

try a tranquilizing tub

Many a weary and depressed person has snapped out of his gloomy mood after soaking in a tranquilizing tub. You will be surprised and gratified at how much it helps to cast off the worries and cares of the day. Always remember this principle of physical medicine: extremes of cold and heat are stimulating, while a tepid bath, around body temperature, is relaxing.

The running water should be about 100 degrees Fahrenheit

since it cools off slightly while entering the tub. So keep the faucet on to hold the temperature constant while you bathe. Stay in for fifteen minutes to a half hour, longer if you wish. You will find that it does you a world of good, and prepares you, both physically and psychologically, for a sound sleep such as you may not have had for months, perhaps years. While the recent development of chemical tranquilizers has done wonders for the mentally ill, I still prescribe the natural tranquilization of the tepid tub bath for the average person who is temporarily fighting windmills.

how to unlax your muscles

With your room properly aerated, and the lights out, slip into bed in comfortable, unconfining night clothing, or in the nude, if that is your preference. Lie on your back, arms at the sides, feet stretched to their full length. Then start the process of relaxation as follows:

1) Flex and extend the toes three times.
2) Rest for a few seconds.
3) Stiffen the legs and stretch them out hard for one minute.
4) Relax completely, as though you were dead tired and your legs heavy enough to press right down through the mattress.
5) With both hands on your stomach, take a deep belly breath, raising your hands with the abdominal wall when it rises as your diaphragm muscle expands.
6) Repeat three times, filling your lungs with each inhalation, and exhaling through your open mouth freely.

You may fall asleep at any time during this process. If you haven't done so, continue with the following:

7) Stretch out your arms at the sides as fully as possible.
8) Unlax and let them flop loosely on the mattress, as you previously did with your legs.
9) Repeat the breathing exercise above, inhaling slowly through your nose, and inflating your lungs to their full capacity with the diaphragm, not using the chest at all.
10) Exhale through your mouth, and repeat the breathing six times.

If you are still awake, you are a confirmed insomniac, and should continue the relaxing process still further, in this way:

11) Wrinkle your forehead and other facial muscles, exaggerating the tensing of each one

12) Relax the muscles of the face and scalp, allowing them to unwind.

13) Repeat the process of tensing and relaxing a half-dozen times.

14) Stiffen your neck muscles, and stretch your neck as far toward the headboard as possible.

15) Relax and repeat six times.

16) Repeat the belly breathing, slowly and rhythmically.

Somewhere during this relaxing process, very likely between items 6 and 10, you should fall asleep without being conscious of having done so. Many of my patients required no further use of sleeping pills after they had learned this tension-easing technique. There is no good reason why you cannot do the same.

Have faith in yourself: in your judgment, your sanity, your will power, and you will find that falling fast asleep is as easy as rolling off a log.

Doc Silvers says: "**Sleep comes to him who seeks it least.**"

Treating Common Skin Disorders
Without Costly Drugs and Cosmetics

12 It is regrettable that we can't go back 50 years or so to the time when patent medicines were in their heyday. Around the turn of the century, newspapers and periodicals were jampacked with advertisements extolling the virtues of a variety of nostrums which were claimed to cure every disease known to mankind, including the killers cancer and consumption. In those days, piddling skin ailments were a pushover. Here is a typical example of an ad for a medicament which cured all skin diseases pronto:

KICKAPOO INDIAN SALVE!

Made from Buffalo Tallow, combined with
Healing Herbs and Barks

It is a perfect cure-all in Skin Diseases—for the various forms of Tetter, dry, scaly, moist or itchy, for Erysipelas, recent or chronic; Pimples or Blotches on the Face, Scald Head, Barber's Itch, and all annoying, unsightly eruptions of the skin; also, painful soft corns, and Burns and Itching Piles. Sold by All Druggists. Price 25 Cents.

This type of advertising got you coming and going, for even if you had the unblemished complexion of Venus, you were pretty certain to be suffering from corns or piles of piles. And since, as Alexander Pope pointed out in his *Essay on Man*, "Hope springs eternal in the human breast," thousands invested a quarter, thus assumedly curing themselves of every skin disease for all time, plus the premium of relief from corns and piles. I don't blame them for a minute. In fact, the advertisement still sounds so convincing that, if Kickapoo Indian Salve were still available, I'd be tempted to try some myself.

While such blatant promotion is rarely observed today—though some vestiges are to be found on radio and television—hope still springs eternal, and the general public spends billions of dollars annually for panaceas as valueless as Kickapoo Indian Salve. As a doctor, I have had many opportunities to observe, in passing, the clutter of cosmetics on the mirrored vanities in my female patients' bedrooms. American women particularly, literally spend a fortune on oils, creams, salves, ointments, lotions, powders, rouge, perfumes and paints. In his classic study, *The Human Face,** John Brophy tells it better than I can:

"Powder, rouge, lipstick, and endless creams are put to work to amend the unsatisfactory complexion. Sometimes little attempt is made to imitate any effect observable in nature, but in general what is aimed at is a similitude of a clear complexion.... The women of Crete, Greece, Egypt, China, and other ancient civilizations are known to have used cosmetics.... Oily and scented unguents, replaced in modern times by skin creams, were applied to soften the texture of the skin and to keep the surfaces of the lips supple. Apple juice (the original 'pomade'), lemon juice, and other acid tinctures were used for whitening the skin, and wealthy beauties have not merely washed but bathed hopefully in milk. Paint was often put on in coats. Many of the Roman satirists direct their criticisms as fiercely against women's toilets as against their morals."

why cosmetics aren't always necessary

To a mere man, and especially to a physician, much of this plethora of cosmetics is a wasteful extravagance. We want our women to be lovely, of course, and whatever means they use to attain beauty is, I suppose, none of our concern. But from my

* Prentice-Hall, Inc., Englewood Cliffs, N.J., 1946.

professional view, if they'd spend some of that money on the proper foods and oils for internal consumption, they would acquire much better complexions.

I'm not going to get up on a soapbox and decry the excessive use of cosmetics. The resultant outcry from womankind would have me licked before I started. However, I will say—and I *do* say—that much of it is valueless.

There is one cosmetic which fulfills 90 percent of a woman's beauty requirements. If, in addition, she wishes to use some powder, a bit of rouge, a smidgin of lipstick, and a touch of perfume here and there, I appreciate that it's done to make her look more desirable to men, and thus ensnare us. And who am I to interfere with the biological urge of nature?

However, women can save money by discarding many of their cosmetics, and putting their faith in the most effective skin oil in the world—good, old fashioned cold cream. This all-purpose oil serves every need for cleansing, protection, and beautification. It keeps the skin young by making it smooth, clear and soft. It also relieves chapping irritation, itching, and sunburn. Here is the standard recipe for cold cream, which I recommend:

Home Rx:
   1 oz. spermaceti
   1 oz. white beeswax (bleached beeswax)
   5 ozs. pressed oil of almond
   20 grs. sodium borate or boraxin
   1½ ozs. strong rose water

Pare the spermaceti and white wax into fine shavings, and melt them together over moderate heat. Add the almond oil. Dissolve the sodium borate or boraxin. Add the rose water. Stir rapidly, or beat with spoon or egg beater, until the mixture becomes soft and creamy.

For those who don't wish to make their own, there are many fine cold creams on the market, some containing approximately the same ingredients. Use the one which tests out best for you. Better yet, ask your pharmacist—not your beauty shop operator—which one he would recommend. Show him the above formula, and tell him that you would like to approximate the standard pharmacopoeia recipe. The cream is applied once a day, usually before bedtime, unless more frequent cleansing and oiling of the skin is desired. Such creams will keep for a reasonable length of time in the refrigerator, and when used will be firmer and feel cool and stimulating.

how to avoid scaly skin

When the skin assumes a scaly appearance like fishskin or alligator hide, the condition is known medically as ichthyosis. The backs of the elbows, outer surfaces of the knees and calves, are the most commonly affected areas. The skin becomes dry, harsh, scaly, and rough, in some instances showing desquamation or peeling of the scales. It develops a sallow and dirty aspect, and is most troublesome in winter and in colder climates.

Applying cold cream, and avoiding soap and other irritants, is beneficial in ordinary cases. A peeling effect may be obtained by adding 30 grains of salicylic acid to the recipe given above, which makes it appreciably more effective for obstinate patches of alligator hide about the elbows and knees. Obstinate cases need medical attention, which would mean delving into the patient's nutritional status, the functioning of the endocrine glands of internal secretion, and might require such physical therapy as hypertonic or alkaline baths, ultraviolet or natural sun baths, and an optimal daily ration of iodine and the sunshine Vitamin D.

Another use for the skin cream, without the salicylic acid, is for neutralizing the effect of soap following a shampoo. Just part the hair, and apply a small amount to the scalp, rubbing it in with the fingertips.

Oil of sesame has been used for centuries as a beauty oil, and is still popular with the Persians and Egyptians. Creams that used to come in a jar are now available in the handier plastic lotion bottles, which protect the contents from air and contamination, and so last longer, besides needing no refrigeration. For dry and itching skin, lanolin and menthol are added to the skin oil, and can be obtained from your pharmacist in already prepared plastic lotion bottles.

The specific vitamin, if there is any such, for dry skin and eyes, is Vitamin A. Great relief from this common condition is obtainable within a short time by the simple procedure of swallowing a capsule of 25,000 units of Vitamin A after breakfast each morning. An interesting effect is that night blindness can often be avoided by this simple technique. So if you have difficulty with your vision at twilight, which is when many auto accidents occur, this dietary supplement will help you.

In practically all of the skin irritations for which oils and lotions are used, the prime cause is too much bathing and washing with strong soaps or other cleansers, the chief factor being the removal of the natural sebum or skin oil. To alleviate this condition, the oil balance must be restored. This holds good for both sexes, and there is no valid excuse for neglecting to help nature perform its normal functions in improving one's looks, disposition, and morale as well. The condition of the skin, it should be noted, has a definite effect upon one's temperament and personality. In proof, we need only note the number of people with skin trouble who are sent by general practitioners and dermatologists to psychiatrists for treatment.

treatment for poison ivy

The *bête noire* (black beast) of outdoor living in the summer months, poison ivy is undoubtedly the most aggravating of allergic skin diseases. Interestingly enough, I have often observed campers innocently exposed, not at camp where there was no sign of the poisonous weed, but alongside a road while changing a tire. The resultant contact dermatitis in the sensitive person can be most frustrating, to say the least, when the skin of the face, arms and legs are all involved.

The specific consists of a special ointment—or better still, lotion —of an antihistaminic with zirconium oxide, which is applied locally over each lesion. Any druggist can supply it. No bandaging should be permitted to irritate and remove the newly formed granulated tissue.

In very severe cases, your doctor will offer some surcease from itching discomfort by application orally, or by injection of a steroid like the improved triamcinolone, which is made synthetically and, in small doses and without side reactions, will relieve all forms of tissue inflammation.

Poison ivy, which in medicalese is grouped with poison oak and poison sumach, can now be prevented by taking small doses of the fluid extract orally. Ask your pharmacist for a two-ounce bottle of *rhus toxicodendrum*, which is put out by Mulford Colloid Laboratories. Start with one drop a day and, if no untoward action occurs, work up to twenty drops. Taken in milk, it has no bitter taste; in fact, it becomes tasteless. Begin this prophylactic treatment early in the spring, and by the time you have used up the extract and are ready to take to the woods, you will be immune from poison ivy for the summer.

An Effective Treatment for Hives

Very often the first symptom of food or drug sensitivity manifests itself in large wheals all over the skin of the body. A wheal consists of a pinpoint red center and a surrounding white area (areola). They may vary in size from a dime to a quarter, depending on the degree of sensitivity. Evidence of eating some new food or taking a new drug is usually evident. Fever is never present. Hives are a form of rash which strikes an otherwise healthy constitution without warning. Many of its victims become unduly frightened, thinking that it is some terrible and incurable disease. However, any doctor will quickly diagnose it and relieve the patient's fears. Usually, he will advise a shot of adrenalin for quick relief. For effective home treatment, ask your pharmacist for an antihistaminic and take as directed. If left alone, hives subside in about ten days.

Home Care for Athlete's Foot

Common athlete's foot (dermatophytosis) is always found between the fourth and fifth toes. These toes are closest together, thus hold moisture longer and, being warmer and less ventilated, are most prone to the vegetative growth which invades the skin at this vulnerable spot. In individuals who are especially sensitive to the fungus, it may spread like a weed, involving any part of the body that offers moisture, warmth, and lack of sunshine. When it invades the skin of the outer ear, it is known as otomycosis, or athlete's ear. The fungus often grows in the crotch under the irritating scrotal supporter, and is spread from there to other parts of the body. The crux of treatment depends on dryness of the area and freedom from irritation.

Borated talcum used early will often stop the spread of this fungoid growth. Undecylenic acid, present in adult sweat, is supplied chemically in ointment, liquid and powder form, by your pharmacist and is highly effective. After cleansing with soap and water, dry the part infected carefully. Apply the powder and keep dry. The liquid form is helpful in cases prone to excessive sweating. The ointment may be applied at night to keep up the action of the acid while sleeping. Remember that you must always dry thoroughly after bathing. Dryness is the *sine qua non* of success in treating this common and irritating disease of the skin.

how to treat burns quickly and effectively

Burns involving large areas of the skin are serious and should be treated by a physician at once. Local burns are best treated by ice-cold applications just as fast as you can get cold water. Ideally, a salt solution made up by adding one teaspoon of common salt to a pint of water, as cold as possible, is applied to the burned area with a saturated piece of sterile gauze. The trick is to get the burn cooled off as fast as possible, and keep it clean of infection.

The application of an ice cube to a small burned area is most effective in relieving pain and preventing the formation of blisters. Some patients of mine who are glass blowers and frequently burn their fingers while at work, grasp their ear lobe with the burned finger. They tell me that the cool lobe quickly cools the burn and usually avoids blistering. The speed with which you apply cold is the important factor. Anesthetic ointments, along with antiseptics, are only required for pain and infection. Open-air treatment without the irritation of a bandage is best. Only your doctor should open any blisters, under sterile precautions, when necessary. Extensive and severe burns require hospitalization, with especial observation for fluid loss and replacement of skin, when required. Always remember that you do the healing yourself, which is Nature's way. What you apply to the burn is primarily for comfort and the pre vention of infection.

What to do about Baldness

There are just two specific "cure-alls"—as the advertisement for Kickapoo Indian Salve would put it—for baldness:

A) Select ancestors with luxuriant hair.

B) Failing that, wear a wig.

While we cannot choose our forebears, we can wear a toupee. However, men, who are most prone to baldness, are hesitant about wearing a toupee to cover a shiny pate. On the other hand, it is interesting and amusing to note that women have worn extra hair for centuries, even though they had plenty of their own. And at this writing, it is fashionable for the ladies to wear wigs atop their own locks of hair. I'm a simple man, so don't ask me why. From the view of the ordinary male, there's never any rhyme or reason for the dictates of feminine fashion. When I'm cornered in a discussion on this subject, I rest my case by falling back on the psychological motivation that female fashion is obviously a prime strategy in woman's eternal pursuit of the male. After that scientific observation, I exit hastily to avoid becoming that not-so-innocent victim of assault and battery.

Let me hasten to add that I have no personal objection to any fashion—that women take up—however absurd it may seem from the male view. Since their intention is to make themselves more attractive, I am happy to be one of their many male admirers. However, from the professional view—if it is possible to separate the doctor from the man—I do criticize a fashion if it appears harmful from the standpoint of good health. And the presently popular wigs *are* detrimental to hair health because they prevent the natural hair and scalp from getting the exposure to sun and air that all skin surfaces require.

Baldness—it should be especially noted by the women in my audience—is of particular concern to women today. That's because, just recently, dermatologists have been noting an increase in the prevalence of baldness amongst women. No longer is it a male condition alone. Authorities estimate that nearly twenty percent of all adult women now have a hair-loss problem, and the prediction is that it will continue to rise in frequency. Therefore, in discussing this subject, I am, in general, addressing both sexes.

A common scalp disease, often associated with baldness, is seborrhoea. It begins with dandruff, or the appearance of a slight gray scaling, accompanied by either oiliness or dryness of the hair. In most instances, the hair tends to become devitalized, and slight or severe baldness may occur. Not infrequently, a relatively mild degree of seborrhoea may result in extensive loss of hair.

Treatment to prevent the spread of this condition includes the restriction of starch, fat, and sugar in the diet, regular physical activity, and plenty of sun and air. Regular hygienic attention should also be given to the scalp and hair. While there is no "pound of cure" for baldness, there are an appreciable number of "ounces of prevention" which can be helpful.

Home Rx:

1) Men: don't wear a hat, unless you feel that you must on such formal occasions as weddings and funerals. Expose your hair and scalp to the elements, even when it rains. In this connection, when I was a lad I was told that if I bared my head in the rain I would grow tall. Well, I followed instructions faithfully, but it didn't add an inch to my growth. Yet though I'm short, it is still good therapy.

2) Women: don't wear tight hats. If you insist on covering your crowning glory, wear one of those adorable little veils which give your scalp a chance to breathe and don't hide the beauty of your hair.

3) Have a shampoo once a week, twice if your hair is oily. Afterwards, wash out the shampoo with Aveeno Soap Cake (which I shall mention in detail later).

4) Brush your hair daily with a soft-bristle brush.

5) Use a comb—one with blunt teeth—as little as possible, for it can injure any delicate new hairs that may be growing in.

6) Massage the scalp daily with the fingertips.

7) Women: Never dress the hair in a tight coiffeur as the constant pulling can bring on baldness at the temples.

8) Don't waste your money on so-called "hair restorative" treatments for they are as worthless as Kickapoo Indian Salve.

9) The moment you notice signs of advancing baldness, consult your doctor or a dermatologist. Remember, once you lose your hair, it is gone forever.

10) If all else fails, wear a wig. While a good one is expensive, today's modern toupee is undetectable.

Doc Silvers says: "While a high forehead has been considered a sign of intelligence, a receding hairline has no such significance."

How to Keep Your Skin Healthy, Clear, and Youthful at Any Age

It was Ben Franklin who said: "In this world, nothing is certain but death and taxes." Another certainty is the process of aging. We inevitably grow older, chronologically and constitutionally, as time ticks the hours away. Every part of our body ages, though, it is interesting to note, not necessarily the mind. The record shows that many people are mentally active throughout life. A few contemporary examples that come to mind are Bernard Baruch, park-bench financier; Pablo Casals, famous cellist; Harry Emerson Fosdick and John Haynes Holmes, spiritual leaders; and the late Frank Lloyd Wright, world-renowned architect.

I have much to say about longevity in this book. In fact, every subject covered is either directly or indirectly concerned with it, which is natural since all aspects of healthful living have an important bearing, in varying degree, upon the length of life, its purposes, accomplishments, and enjoyment. At this point, however, we are expressly concerned with the aging of the skin.

In recent years, because of the progressive aging of the population, medical research has devoted more and more study to the field of geriatrics, which is concerned with the problems and diseases of aging and old age. One of the findings is that chronological and biological age are not necessarily comparable. Another, of interest to everyone since we all grow older, is that the visible signs of aging—which heretofore had been accepted as inevitable—can be delayed, and sometimes even avoided.

And so it is with the skin; it ages, naturally, but age and the condition of the skin are not always comparable. Some young folk may, due to poor hygienic care, have a skin that appears old. On the other hand, some older folk may have a skin sufficient in oil, secreted by the sebaceous glands, to keep it pliant, soft, and youthful looking.

Speaking in general terms, in youth the skin is moist and oily, while in aging it gets dry and rough, harsh and scaly. The cleansing and treatment of the skin, therefore, depends upon its present condition; what is good for it in youth is bad for it in middle age, and vice versa.

When you're young, you can be liberal with soap and water. Any toilet soap is indicated for the oily skin of acne, so prevalent among teenagers, in washing off the excess natural skin oil. For the mature, however, whose skin lacks essential oils, the use of ordinary soap should be avoided as it depletes the oil needed to keep the skin moist, slightly greasy, clear and smooth. Regular soap also frequently causes severe itching (pruritus) on older skin. We thus reach two conclusions:

A) It is unwise for the young to use any creams, or oily, greasy cosmetics.

B) It is a mistake for the mature to use soap and water on the skin.

The skin is normally on the acid side, which is why damage to the mature skin can be occasioned by excessive soaping. A bland oil, such as olive, almond, or sesame, is recommended. In addition, the cold cream previously given should be used daily.

For tub baths, I prescribe Aveeno Oilated, available in 10-ounce cans, and obtainable at all druggists. It is a super-oiled colloidal oatmeal concentrate, impregnated with liquid petrolatum and a special hypo-allergenic fraction of lanolin. This colloidal, emollient bath soothes and relieves delicate, sensitive, or itching skin, and also lubricates and softens taut, dry skin.

Home Rx: Aveeno Oilated
   Adults—3 to 4 rounded tablespoons
   Children—1 to 2 rounded tablespoons
   Babies—2 to 3 level teaspoons

Add required amount of Aveeno Oilated to a tub of warm water (103 degrees F.) and stir well. Use just enough water to cover the body. Bathe for 10 to 20 minutes, as desired.

Aveeno Oilated also comes in a soap cake, which has a sudsy, oily action, and is moderately priced. For dry or itchy skin, take the tub bath twice a week. Alternate with the soap cake on face and hands for persistent dryness and irritation.

The epidermis is constantly being shed and replaced. The ring around the bathtub, no matter how clean your skin may be, is telltale evidence of the shedding skin, which clings so tenaciously to the porcelain. A deeper layer, called the dermis, is where the new skin cells are constantly being formed, ready to replace the old cells sloughing off on the surface. Because of this continuous process, the aging skin, which has less natural oil, benefits from the hygienic and therapeutic treatment of colloidal emollient baths.

The skin of older folk gives more trouble in winter, and it is not because of cold weather. Lack of moisture in our overheated homes produces the same effect upon the skin as it does on book bindings, musical instruments, furniture, and growing plants. In the winter season, it is most important that aging skin get its daily ration of oil and cold cream to keep it in a more supple condition. Properly regulated air conditioning is also helpful. Lacking that, the evaporation of a couple of gallons of water daily in heated rooms in order to supply needed moisture is an effective means of avoiding damage to aging skin.

Constipation is often made the goat for skin abnormalities. Many people who have an unclear skin, and are also troubled with constipation, reason that the former is caused by the latter. They thereupon take laxatives in an effort to improve the condition of their skin. However, laxatives do not solve this distressing problem.

Constipation is an all-too-common disorder, which is considered by some medical authorities to be the disease of civilization. Millions of Americans eat laxatives like candy. In fact, some *are* candy-coated. Taking laxatives regularly is a dangerous habit, and you should never use them, except upon occasion, unless they are prescribed by your family doctor.

Should you be the victim of the mineral oil habit—and since old Doc Lane of England started this foolish and harmful craze years ago, many of us are—you are doing yourself more damage than good by depending on it.

Mineral oil retards digestion by coating the particles of food eaten, thus interfering with the absorption of the products of the resultant poorer digestive process. It also interferes with the absorption of minerals, especially such important ones as calcium and phosphorus. In addition, mineral oil prevents the reabsorption of bile from the intestine, thereby curtailing biliary and pancreatic enzymatic action. And since both vitamins A and D, like K and E, are all fat soluble, it prevents their normal utilization.

Today we know that vegetable oils can be substituted to great advantage, if taken in recommended dosages. A large dose of any vegetable oil is laxative in action, and has no harmful side effects. So if you've been taking mineral oil for constipation, discontinue its use immediately, and switch to a vegetable oil of your choice as an occasional purgative. If you should suffer from chronic constipation, see your physician without further delay.

treating pimples and boils

While pimples pop up more frequently in the young, they may appear at any age. Fortunately, the indicated home treatment is simple and effective. Just as soon as you note the onset of a pimple, apply iodine locally and repeatedly during the first twenty-four hours. As a rule, you will be rewarded by the disappearance of the infection and inflammation in a matter of a few days, with no surgery required. This has occurred so frequently in my patients over the years that I pass it on to you for your convenience and benefit.

Should there be an infection on the face above the upper lip, avoid surgery until you have completely softened and encircled, or walled off, the mass. This procedure is important because the drainage from the abscess might reach the brain via the angular veins of the nose and into the cavernous sinus at its base. Never squeeze a pimple which is above the level of the upper lip. Always apply hot compresses until it comes to a white head, and is completely sealed off from the surrounding tissue. Then if it is cut open carefully, it will drain freely to the exterior, and not spread upward toward the brain.

Most people, both young and old, have experienced, upon occasion, the devilish pain of a boil. However, the suffering is needless, for this superficial infection can be controlled and absorbed with little discomfort and no surgical interference, if treated immediately upon its appearance.

Home Rx:

1) Apply copious swabbings of tincture of iodine to the incipient boil for one minute.

2) Repeat morning and night; every four hours for those with tough skins.

Within 40 hours, the swelling disappears, and pus formation and surgical drainage are avoided. The advantage of this simple technique is that it can be safely used at home on any area, even such places as the back of the neck, where the infection cannot be spotted by direct vision but must be located by touch. This method is sure-fire, as I well know from experience, for whenever I wear a starched collar, and microscopically abrade the skin on the back of my neck, a boil invariably rears its painful head. But the application of iodine turns the trick every time.

how to treat and protect minor skin injuries

Fresh skin injuries should first be cleansed with peroxide or tincture of green soap, and then allowed to air dry. Often you can do away with a bandage by the application of phenolated calamine solution, available from your pharmacist. At children's camp, where skin abrasions keep the nurse busy, we get the best results by allowing drying in the sun before the above solution is swabbed on with a cotton applicator. The injury is again permitted to dry, and is then kept free of covering until the scab comes off. Only in the case of a bleeding wound is a bandage used with pressure under sterile precautions. The lack of bandage is because I have found, in my lengthy camp experience, that wounds heal much faster, and with more freedom from pustulation. Every time you remove a bandage, you take off the new granulation with the gauze, thereby forcing nature to repeat its effort to heal a break in the skin. Without a bandage, you also get more oxygen to the cut or abrasion, so diminishing the chance of tetanus developing in the wound. Tetanus germs live only in the absence of oxygen, which is why a punctured wound is so much more dangerous.

Another unusual and most helpful method for increasing the healing of the skin, while protecting it against the outer elements, is by the application of egg white. Remove the white from a fresh egg, previously having scalded it to make certain that no infectious material is clinging to the shell. The wound must be clean, and the egg white sterile before it is applied. The egg white dries and seals the wound, allowing it to heal with a minimum of disturbance to the formation of the granulation tissue. In addition, the rich supply of protein applied locally hastens the otherwise more sluggish healing process. During my summers as a camp physician, I have used this technique frequently, even for such slow-healing wounds as bed sores, and have always obtained gratifying results. *Never* coat a punctured wound, no matter how clean the surface, for you are thereby aiding any anaerobic organisms (those which grow in the absence of oxygen) like tetanus, which may be present. For many years, I have insisted that every child get a booster shot against tetanus before coming to camp each summer, and thus far I have never encountered this infectious disease.

how your skin reflects your general health

Remember that what you put on your skin is never as important as what you feed it. What goes into your skin depends upon many factors. What you eat and drink, and what you take in the form of medicine, are of primary importance. Your sensitive skin is an accurate barometer of your kind of life. In addition to these basics, you can treat your skin from the outside as well as the inside. As you get older, shun ordinary soaps, and give your skin the complete home care, as I have suggested, that it deserves. In doing so, you will retard, and may even avoid, the aging appearance of your skin.

I am sure you have seen, as I have, old, and even elderly, people, who have retained the healthy, clear, smooth complexion of their younger days. Medical science now knows that many of the evidences of aging can be slowed down and minimized, if not entirely obliterated. A number of the finest looking men and loveliest looking women I know are getting on in years. They continue to have attractive complexions because they treat their bodies, inside and out, with respect. And, too, it may also be the outward expression of the beauty of their souls.

Doc Silvers says: "Take good care of your skin, for it is the one garment that, throughout life, you never remove."

How to Avoid Nose Ailments

13
I previously waxed nostalgic about "the good old days" when sure-fire cures were sold for just about every disease known to man, including cancer, tuberculosis, and drug addiction. Many of them had quite a kick, containing, as they did, copious quantities of alcohol. Parker's True Tonic, for example, which was supposed to cure alcoholism, was found to be generously spiked—over 40%—with alcohol. And although, a half-century later, we still have no cure for the common cold, this universal infection, which annually lays millions low, was a pushover for the "medicine men" of that day, as witness this advertisement:

WHITE BEAVER'S COUGH CREAM
HEALS DISEASED LUNGS AND CURES COUGHS
AND COLDS
Made only by Dr. (sic) Frank Powell, Medicine Chief of the
Winnebago Indians, La Crosse, Wis. Sold by all druggists.

The concerted efforts of the American Medical Association, ethical drug manufacturers, and the better newspapers and magazines, banned that kind of "come on" long ago. Meanwhile, we continue to get chills and fever, and sniffle and sneeze, come fall until spring. There are, however, a number of effective ways of preventing a cold from occurring in the first place. All we need do is take the proper precautions.

Psychologically, the trouble with prevention is that it isn't as dramatic as a cure. When your doctor pulls you through a bout with some disease, your illness becomes a statistical fact, and is duly entered in the record books. But if, for example, in the course of a year, by using preventive measures, you avoid, let's say, three colds, two ear infections, one boil, and four cases of athlete's foot, there is no way of your knowing it, so it cannot be recorded. All you can say is that you have felt better during those 12 months. However, you have, in this instance, actually avoided ten illnesses, which would not be at all unusual, and can easily be done by anyone, year in and year out, by sidestepping infection and injury and, should they occur, taking the necessary steps to relieve or abort them.

how your nose governs other body functions

Anatomically, the nose is the drainage basin for the four pairs of sinuses. Their purpose is to lighten the weight of the skull, so making less work for the neck muscles, and they also afford resonance to our voices. The daily sinus secretion from all four pairs is approximately one pint. Add to this the quart of saliva secreted by the salivary glands each day, and you will appreciate the efficient way in which our mucus membranes are kept constantly moist. Never expectorate unless you must as it wastes the benefits of these bountiful secretions. Not only do they protect our mouth and gastrointestinal (stomach and bowel) canal by lubrication, but they also contain natural immunizing agents which guard us against infections.

Physiologically, the nose is the "air conditioner" of the body. It warms, moistens, and cleans by filtering the air before it passes through the larynx and the lungs. It may be of interest to note here how this human air-conditioning system is adapted for the Eskimo living in the frozen tundras of the arctic. His nose is narrow, and his nostrils are just slits to allow as little of the freezing air into his lungs as possible before it is warmed, moistened, and filtered by the nasal spongy masses called the turbinates. On the other hand, the nose of the native who lives in a moist, tropical climate, is wide and the nostrils distended, as he doesn't need the protection from an adverse environment, as does the Eskimo. This is yet another example of Nature's many wonders: the adaptation to one's environment.

The turbinates on each side of the nasal wall divide the nasal cavity into three channels, called the inferior, middle, and superior nasal meati (passages). The surprising thing is that the drainage is actually uphill, against the force of gravity. Small, hairlike appendages called cilia, propel the mucus upward toward its exit into the middle meatus. Knowing this, we understand why proper drainage from the sinuses is assisted by bending the head forward into the lap while in a seated position.

treatment of sinus infection and headache

Sinus infection and the resultant headache is best relieved in the acute stage, during the first forty-eight hours, that is, with an ice-cold compress dipped into a cold hypertonic salt solution. The Rx was given in an earlier chapter, but I am repeating it here for your convenience.

Home Rx:
  1 tablespoon epsom salt
  1 teaspoon bircarbonate of soda
  1 pint ice-cold water

Dip a compress or small towel into the solution, wring out the excess and, with your head bent down to your lap, apply over the sinuses. After 48 hours, when the condition becomes subacute (reduced), change to compresses of the same solution which are as hot as you can tolerate them, reimmersing them when they cool off. Continue this therapy for a quarter-hour, twice a day, three times if the pain is severe.

Should the nasal passages be obstructed, you may shrink the swollen blood vessels with a spray of any of the numerous products on the market such as Neo-Synephrine 1%, privine, or biomydrin. Don't, however, continue the use of a tissue-shrinking nasal spray or tampons any longer than absolutely necessary. Prolonged use of these vasoconstrictors of the nasal turbinates results in rhinitis medicamentosa (inflammation of the inner nasal tissues) as a side effect of the treatment. Remember that *only* in the acute stage of nasal turbinate swelling is it advisable to use a shrinking solution or nasal spray. It may be of interest to you to note here that Newton's third law of motion, "Every action has an equal and opposite reaction," also holds true for our nasal structures. Because of it, the relief afforded by the temporary vasoconstriction is later, in about two hours, followed up by a reaction which swells up the obstruction again; and there you are, right back where you started. So be guided by Isaac Newton, and you won't go wrong.

Help for Hay Fever

Sensitivity to any substance may produce a characteristic reaction. Some manifest it in the nose and throat or the bronchial tubes; others who are allergic show its effects on the skin or intestinal tract. Pollinosis is the medical term for hay fever. If it is due to grasses or trees, it will trouble you only in the early spring and summer; but if you are sensitive to ragweed, and you live in the East, your troubles begin in the middle of August and last up to the first frost.

Home Rx:

The eyes, nose and throat, as a rule, get the brunt of the effect of the pollen. For the eyes, a mild wash two or three times a day is most helpful. Mix one teaspoonful of boric acid powder in eight ounces of water; boil for a few minutes and allow to cool before using. Use an eyecup and lave away any of the irritating pollen that may have gotten into your eyes. Estivin is obtainable from your druggist and aids in relieving the itching and smarting. Put two drops into each eye three times a day. Antihistaminics are most helpful for temporary relief, though desensitization by your doctor is a more permanent treatment. Nose drops should be used only according to necessity as they become habit-forming and do damage to the nasal mucosa. For temporary relief only, get one-half percent of Neo-Synephrine in a one-ounce dropper bottle from your pharmacist. Put two drops into each nostril every four hours.

Make sure to throw your head all the way back so that none of the medication gets into the Eustachian tubes, which thereby might carry an infection to the ears.

Treatment for Smoker's Drip

The common drip from behind the nasal cavities, of which all smokers complain, is the result of the drying and thickening of the normal sinus secretion as it courses down the channel between the back of the nose (naso-pharynx) and the throat (oropharynx). The thickened mucous secretion catches hold on the mucosa of the back of the throat and hangs on tenaciously. Severe hawking will eventually dislodge the globus (lump) and the smoker is relieved until it forms again. For this condition, washing of the nasal cavities is helpful.

Home Rx:

1 level teaspoon of salt
1 pint of warm water

While douching the nasal cavity, keep your head bent forward to avoid forcing the fluid into the ear canals via the Eustachian tubes. Please do not confuse this natural salt solution with the hypertonic salt solution mentioned elsewhere as they are not the same, and serve different purposes. The only sure cure for this retronasal tickle and the resultant cough is to stop smoking cigarettes entirely. If you have the determination to do so, you will never regret it.

You Can Avoid Colds

I have already gone out on a limb and stated categorically that the incidence of common ailments can be reduced 50% or more by the observance of preventive measures. I'll even go farther than that. In some thirty years as a camp physician, my experience with and observation of children leads me to the firm conclusion that illness amongst them is directly or indirectly due to *preventable* respiratory infections in *at least 75%* of all cases!

Whether this high percentage of prevention holds true for adults as well has not been statistically determined. But all of the facts and figures lead to the conclusion that afflictions common to the adult population can be reduced appreciably. If you can cut in half the number of colds you usually have in a year, I am sure you will agree that it is well worth the little time and trouble it takes to accomplish that end. And you might very well reduce them even further. In fact, if you are careful in safeguarding yourself against exposure, you may have no colds at all!

what you need to know about colds

In order to prevent or treat a cold, we should, first of all, know what it is. A cold is man's most prevalent affliction. The principal reason it is so common is that it is contagious. You can't catch a cold out of the clear blue sky; you have to get it from someone who already has a cold. All methods of prevention are based on that fact alone, so please keep it in mind.

A cold is a catarrhal infection of the nose and upper air passages or a common respiratory infection. Today we know that it is due to a filterable virus, which is frequently accompanied by such other germs as staphylococci, pneumococci, and streptococci. Very likely you have wondered why medical science hasn't yet developed a vaccine for the prevention of colds. But once you know the extent of the problem, you readily understand the reason, which is that there is such a wide variety of viruses that no one vaccine can cover them all. If there were just a single type of germ to contend with, the problem would be immensely simplified, and the common cold could be conquered in short order.

You have undoubtedly heard the witticism which says that when a cold is treated, it lasts two weeks, and when it is not treated, it lasts only 14 days. While this is amusing, it doesn't jibe with the facts. A cold usually starts in the nose. However, if it is not treated, complications set in. It may spread to the sinuses, the Eustachian tubes, middle ears, pharynx, larynx, and on to the trachea (windpipe), bronchi, and lungs. Treatment, therefore, is most important in stopping the progress of the malady. Thus there is a twofold purpose involved: use preventive measures to avoid catching cold; and if you do get one, treat it immediately to minimize its effect.

How to Prevent Colds

1) First of all, maintain your body's resistance to infection by normal living, with an adequate diet, regular exercise, and enough rest. That's basic. While some contagious diseases cannot be warded off by a strong constitution, it is definitely known that a high resistance is effective, at least to some degree, in avoiding the occurrence of colds.

2) Insofar as possible, when colds are prevalent, keep out of crowds. While I don't propose that you should become a hermit and live in isolation on a hilltop, there are a number of precautionary measures you can take in this respect which will definitely reduce the incidence of infection.

a) When you go to a movie, select a seat away from the crowd. And if someone nearby should start sneezing or coughing, immediately get up and move away.

b) If you have a dinner date or some other engagement, should any member of the party have a cold, do not hesitate to cancel the date pronto. Don't be concerned about being considered a spoilsport. Remember, in all things, your health comes first, and if you explain to your relatives and friends that it is a most important health measure, I am sure that they will understand. I know a couple who observe this rule religiously, and they have told me that, while they used to get three or four colds a year, now they rarely have one. "The only exception we make," they say with a smile, "is for weddings and funerals."

c) If you work in an office, when some other member of the staff has a cold, instead of communicating with him or her directly, use the interoffice phone.

d) If you must associate with someone with a cold, keep yourself at least four feet away. Should he start to sneeze, immediately cover your nose and mouth with your own handkerchief.

e) In a public conveyance, if a passenger near you sneezes or coughs, protect yourself with your handkerchief and then take a seat elsewhere.

f) Since an infection often occurs through the nose, if you can't avoid being close to someone with a cold, place cotton stopples in your nostrils and breathe through your mouth until you can manage to get away. Though not a sure preventive, it will afford you at least some protection.

3) Keep comfortably warm and dry. While low temperatures and wet feet will not give you a cold—you have to catch it from someone, remember—they may lower your natural immunity and thus make you more susceptible to infection.

4) "Do unto others as you would that they should do unto you," is the Golden Rule. When you have a cold, isolate yourself from others as much as possible so that you won't be a "Typhoid Mary" and infect them. In my work with children at camp, I have found that isolation is the *sine qua non*, indispensable, that is, to success in keeping to an absolute minimum the incidence of colds. As soon as a camp counsellor notes that a youngster has any beginning symptoms of a cold, such as a stuffy nose, sore throat, hoarseness or cough, he is referred to me at the infirmary for a checkup and, if so indicated, is isolated at once. An interesting observation in this connection is that counsellors who are six feet or more in height, thus towering over the children, are much less prone to spray infection. As for myself, in my daily tasks in the field of nose and throat therapy, I use a transparent mask which I devised some forty years ago. In wearing it, I can sit right up close to the patient while the film separates us, and our conversational spray is caught on the plastic mask which is attached to my head mirror and stands away from my face, so allowing for ventilation and comfort. Thus I don't catch my patient's cold and, should I have one, he or she isn't infected with mine.

5) Ask your doctor about the advisability of having yourself immunized against influenza types A & B and the Asian variety. While these shots won't cure the common cold, they may well abort more serious complications. I have them each year, prior to the camp season, and rarely lose a day from my activities all summer long.

Home Rx for Colds

In combating the common cold, the front line of defense is to use the various means of prevention that have been suggested. If, unfortunately, you catch a cold nevertheless—frequently the infection is due to someone nearby unexpectedly sneezing without using a handkerchief—you then fall back to the second line of defense and use the following procedure to minimize the extent of the illness and thus avoid complications which would put you out of action for some time.

1) At the very first characteristic signs of a cold: stuffy nose, sore throat, hoarseness or a cough, use quinine medication. Take a two-grain pill every four hours, followed by a hot drink consisting of the juice of half a lemon, two tablespoons of honey, and 200 mg. of Vitamin C, in a glass of boiled water. While this medication won't kill the invading organisms, it does prevent their multiplication, and your immune-producing lymph-adenoid cells do the rest for your protection. Quinine, by the way, used to be standard treatment during the early stage of a cold, but in the past quarter-century or so, its value has been neglected. But quinine is still definitely helpful in the early treatment of the common cold, and I advise it. However, do not take larger doses than prescribed above as they may result in dizziness, ringing of the ears, and contraction of the uterus in pregnancy.

2) Go to bed at once, and stay there for twenty-four hours. If it is during the work week, it is better to take one day off rather than wait until the cold is severe, when you may have to be away from your employment for several days, perhaps even a week.

3) Take a hot mustard foot bath, using one or two tablespoons of mustard dissolved in a vessel of hot water. It is of benefit, whether or not you sweat. The mustard bath acts by drawing blood away from the head and upper part of the torso to the feet and skin surface. When sweating does occur, you may be breaking a fever, or it may be an indication of the effectiveness of the treatment. Copious sweating affords relief, whether or not you get rid of any toxins via the skin. Don't worry about drafts after this therapy; just make yourself comfortable in bed and remain at rest.

4) If you do not cough, drink lots of water and/or fruit juice. However, if your cold is complicated by a cough, you will have less throat discomfort and tickle if you avoid cold drinks. Instead, take hot drinks, which are more soothing and stimulate more goblet (mucus-secreting) cell action, thus keeping the throat moist, and, therefore, less irritated. Hot drinks are also indicated for older folk who are not as vigorous as they used to be. Hot lemonade with honey, milk, chocolate, soup, or other wholesome beverages served hot, are all beneficial.

5) Eat sensibly, and avoid overeating and too hasty swallowing of food before it is thoroughly masticated as this causes liver congestion and subsequent embarrassment of the circulation with swelling of the nasal and sinus vessels. Your head will feel full and heavy, and your nostrils completely obstructed, as a result of this vascular congestion. Should this condition transpire, a nasal spray is indicated, which, with its vaso-constrictor action, will establish ventilation for about four hours.

6) If you have a fever and discomfort is intolerable, you may take aspirin. I always advise an alkali with the aspirin to buffer it. Use milk of magnesia in tablet form, if constipated; bicarbonate of soda if not.

7) To help relieve congestion, rub camphorated oil, or a menthol and camphor mixture, over the bridge of the nose, and on the throat and chest. Use just enough to thinly coat the skin. In this connection, please note that, in the case of an infant, camphor must be very carefully applied. Should some accidentally get on the garment, it can become toxic to a baby, if left alone to breathe it for several hours.

8) Smoking is contraindicated during the course of a cold as it definitely aggravates the symptoms. Therefore, if you are a smoker, curtail your consumption of cigarettes or, better yet, cut them out entirely until you are well again.

How to Blow Your Nose

Right off, I suppose you'll say that you already know now to blow your nose; after all, you've been doing it for years. Be that as it may, in my long medical practice, I have rarely encountered anyone who really knew how to blow his nose to the best and safest effect. The simple technique of blowing your nose is most important when it comes to preventing the ascent of a nose and throat infection into the tubes back of the nose, which lead to the middle ears. There are many wrong methods, but only one right way to blow your nose. Follow these instructions, and you will help avoid an unnecessary ear infection.

1) Drop your head forward, with your eyes looking down at the floor, before you begin to blow.

2) Do not obstruct the nostrils by pinching them or contracting them with your handkerchief. Keep it well away from immediate contact with your nose. The principle which applies here is not to offer obstruction to the nasal outlet.

3) When you blow, keep your mouth wide open.

4) Blow gently and steadily in order to drain the nose freely and not send out the secretion forcefully.

5) Obstructing the nostrils, holding the head erect, closing the mouth and blowing with force, may not only cause congestion of the middle ear, or one or more of the sinuses, but actually force the infection into one of these accessory cavities, causing middle-ear disease, mastoiditis, or even acute sinusitis. Therefore, the least possible amount of nose blowing is always preferable. When you are uncomfortable and must blow your nose, do so easily and gently, with minimum force.

Doc Silvers says: "**Keep your nose, the 'air conditioner' of your body, operating properly, just as you do the air conditioner in your home, and you will have fewer repair bills for both systems.**"

How to Prevent and
Treat Sore Throats

14   When you are troubled by such common throat ailments as a cough, soreness, dryness or hoarseness, you usually reach for some soothing, but narcotic, cough medicine, and I don't blame you. However, it isn't the best thing for the condition, and I don't recommend it. Your cough is Nature's means of getting rid of irritating accumulations. Therefore, the purpose of any medication for a cough should be to loosen up the secretions, and increase Nature's defenses by greater secretion of the goblet cells of the mucous membrane of the nose and throat.

how to make your own cough medicine

A sedative is indicated in only one type of cough, the hacking, nonproductive kind which is harassing and of no physical purpose. This worthless and irritating hack is rarely due to the accumulation of mucus secretion of mostly dead bacteria, which makes it necessary for you to swallow or expectorate. It is, instead, caused as a rule by dryness and congestion of the mucosa back of the throat and nose, where the adenoid shelf is located. Thus what you need is application of a hygroscopic (moisture-holding) solution to the dry area at the back of the throat, so alleviating the tickle which brings on the unproductive cough.

Home Rx:

Silvers' Swab Solution

Resublimed iodine crystals	0.1
Potassium iodide	3.0
Sol. guaiacol	5.0
Essence peppermint	1.0
Honey or glycerine q. s.	100.0

Present this prescription to your pharmacist, and he will make it up for you. When swabbed on the mucous membranes of mouth and throat, the relief is so rapid that coughing is quickly alleviated. The local antisepsis also keeps those you associate with from acquiring what you have when you speak to them, so it works both ways. Dip an applicator into this solution, and swab your sore throat with it three or four times a day. The highly antiseptic effect of the iodine and the guaiacol act together to wash out and destroy the bacterial invaders. In many summers at camp, the use of my throat swab has kept down the spread of infection in children to an absolute minimum, and has also avoided the passing of infection from the upper to the lower respiratory tract, thus keeping the ailment simple, easy to treat, and so hastening recovery.

There are two indicated treatments for a sore throat. My own foolproof cough syrup has aided my patients for years.

Home Rx:

Lemon juice	1 tablespoon
Honey	2 tablespoons (glycerin for diabetics)
Aspirin	1 tablet
Boiled hot water	8 oz. glass

Mix until the aspirin is dissolved. When cool enough for comfort use first as a gargle to rinse out any debris which may have accumulated in your throat, and expectorate. After the initial gargle, gargle again very gently, and then swallow. This lubricates the parched areas, and gives immediate relief to the harassing cough.

This treatment may be repeated, according to necessity, every three to four hours for several days. The gargle provides not only local soothing of the back of your throat, but also the gentle diuretic effect of promoting your kidney secretion, the stimulation of sweating, and the mildly sedative expectorant which loosens and liquefies, thus easing the spasms of coughing. In addition, the citric acid in the lemon juice turns alkaline, and so opposes any acidity which may arise from the infection and fever.

If you should get what is termed "speaker's sore throat," with a raspy voice and accompanying hoarseness, use the same medicament, but make it up in double strength, increasing everything but the hot water. First gargle, and then swallow, as before. The resultant moistening of the mucus membrane, the astringent effect of the lemon juice, and the swallowing after the initial gargle, will, after a rest from speaking, bring your voice back to normal.

Just ordinary gargling by itself is of minimal value as the medicament rarely reaches further than the uvula or front of the throat. Hence, it is the swallowing, rather than the gargle, which is most beneficial. As I remarked before with regard to my throat swab, gargling, like throat swabbing, can be altruistic in that it tends to prevent the spread of your throat infection to others in your immediate vicinity.

Never neglect a sore throat. Even a mild case may be caused by a highly potent organism which could do damage to the heart valves. There are adults who suffer from a heart ailment which, back in childhood, might have been caused by a supposedly innocent throat infection. A culture of the throat is always indicated when a blood-dissolving organism is suspected, and we now culture all organisms to make certain that the proper medication is prescribed. Therefore, if a sore throat persists for more than a few days, consult your family physician.

Medication for Laryngitis

Any infection of the nose and throat may extend downward into the voice box. Public speakers, clergymen, professional singers, teachers, and those who smoke heavily, are particularly prone to the hoarseness which accompanies inflammation of the vocal chords.

Should your hoarseness be due to an infection, it will generally run a course of a week or two before all signs of speech difficulty are eliminated. However, if it continues after you have used the following remedies, then professional medical attention is called for.

Rest is the best treatment for any inflammation, including laryngitis. Communicate via sign language, or by writing on a pad, for just one day, and the next morning you will find that your speaking voice has greatly improved.

Steam inhalations are most beneficial and should be practiced three times a day. Inhale the steam carefully as it comes from the spout of your tea kettle. Keep a foot or so away from the kettle to avoid burning your face. For greater convenience and safety, purchase one of the reasonably priced vaporizers available at all drugstores.

Half a teaspoon of salt mixed into a glass of hot boiled water is an effective rinse for clearing the attached mucus from both nose and throat. Allow to cool a bit to a comfortable temperature and, throwing the head back, instill a few drops of this solution into your nostrils to clean out any accumulations of mucoid material which are obstructing your breathing. As a rinse, it will clear the surface of the throat of mucinous patches. For an excellent gargle, use my homemade cough syrup, given earlier in this chapter, dissolving two aspirins into the mixture instead of one. Expectorate the first mouthful, then gargle and swallow. Repeat three times a day as long as required.

Since the nose is your air conditioner, make certain that it is always open to the free passage of air. The warming, moistening and filtering function of the nose is essential at all times, and particularly when the larynx is affected.

Treatment for Trench Mouth

Infectious gingivitis is the medical term for trench mouth. It is characterized by spongy, raw and bleeding gums, showing a whitish coating surrounded by a red rim (areola). A common cause is unclean dishes used in crowded surroundings, such as a military encampment. Prevention is possible by thorough sterilization of all kitchen utensils, dishes and glassware by washing in boiling water with a soap or detergent.

Home Rx:

Dissolve a teaspoonful of perborate of soda in a glass of boiled water. When cooled down, use as a mouth wash and gargle. Obtain a one-ounce bottle of 2% gentian violet from your druggist. Soak a cotton applicator and cover the gums thoroughly with the gentian violet; allow to dry for about ten minutes. Then chew some sulphathiazole gum, also obtainable at your pharmacist without prescription. This treatment will ordinarily clean up the infection within a few days.

How to Avoid Halitosis

A normally healthy mouth and nose give off no objectionable odor. However, when the gums or mucosa (membranes) of the mouth, or the lining of the nasal cavity, develop an infection, a fetid odor usually ensues. Halitosis, an unpleasant smelling breath, is present only in the abnormal nose and mouth, though, as everyone knows, it often follows the eating of such condiments as onion and garlic. Rarely does a gastric condition give off a foul odor, and then only in serious ailments.

Home Rx:

For the relief of halitosis due to an infection of the buccal mucosa (mouth membranes), dissolve one teaspoonful of aromatized sodium perborate in a half glass of warm water. Rinse the mouth morning and evening after your meal. Allow the action of the medication to remain on the mucous membranes as long as possible. Avoid hard bristles on your toothbrush, and brush your teeth carefully so as not to injure the mucosa of the mouth and gums.

How to Clear up Canker Sores

A common minor, yet nevertheless irritating, ailment that causes pain and discomfort in chewing and swallowing is canker sores.

They consist of inflamed areas along the sides of the mouth or tongue, usually no larger than pinheads. Several theories have been advanced for their formation, but the particular condition most commonly associated with them is hypersensitivity or allergy to some particular food. At times, they may be accompanied by a gastro-intestinal upset. Often no demonstrable illness can be detected.

Locally, the application of Silvers' Solution on a cotton applicator will hasten the absorption and healing process and curb infection. Antihistaminics are helpful where sensitivity exists; ask your druggist for a dozen antihistamine tablets. One tablet should be taken every four hours for several days. Gradual disappearance of the redness and swelling will be noted. If the condition is very stubborn apply an applicator saturated with Silvers' Solution directly to each sore, three times a day after meals. A soothing rinse with a teaspoon of perborate of soda to a glass of warm water will help to cleanse the affected area and hasten healing of the sores.

Are Tonsils Necessary?

Early in this century, it was often customary to have children's tonsils removed on a wholesale basis. A group of mothers would gather their children in one home and await the doctor. When he arrived, he placed the youngsters, one at a time, on the dining-room table and started snipping away. Sometimes he would remove the adenoids, too, without extra charge. By pooling their offspring in this way, the mothers got the job done at what we would today call a discount price.

At that time, it was the prevalent opinion among the laity that tonsils were as unnecessary as the vermiform appendix, though that surgery didn't become fashionable until later. Today, however, we know that your tonsils are an asset to you as they are the center of the immunological—base of immunity, that is—system of the body. Therefore, it is preferable, if possible, to keep your tonsils for your lifetime.

The problem of the tonsils is still with us, though it is not nearly as acute as in the generations before the physiology of the lymphoid tissues of the body was understood. Nowadays, it is unnecessary to remove the entire tonsil by radical means, if the infected crypts are rendered harmless. With the use of electrosurgery—a field in which I specialize—the crypts of the tonsils can be completely opened and drained by performing what I call a diathermo-cryptectomy. This bloodless surgery constitutes a permanent form of drainage for each of the tonsillar crypts. If enlarged, the tonsils can be shrunken by subcoagulation doses of surgical diathermy.

My own experience over a period of 40 years with the management of this tonsillar problem has made hundreds of my patients good friends as well. Many of them have told me that they noticed relief of general bodily pains soon after the fourth or fifth treatment with electrocoagulation. The explanation I have to offer is that the germs imbedded in the infected tonsillar crypts are cremated by the penetrating heat of the resistance of the tissue to the passing of the high frequency current; and the absorption of the end products of these dead bacteria and viruses acts as an autogenous vaccine, made and cultured from your own organisms. It is as though, with each treatment, you were receiving shots of a vaccine made from your own specific infection. This is the same effect, you will remember, as the cold quartz light therapy mentioned earlier.

Should Tonsils be Removed?

Naturally, if they are diseased, the answer is in the affirmative. However, since, as we have seen, they perform a most important bodily function, they should not be excised unless, and until, it is absolutely necessary.

Over the years, many mothers have brought their little children to me for my opinion as to the desirability of removal of their tonsils. They usually come early in the spring, and the anxious mother relates how Jimmy or Nancy has been down with one cold after another, and was frequently absent from school during the winter months.

These youngsters are usually in nursery school or kindergarten, where, for the first time, they come in contact with newer viruses to which we all must develop our own active immunity. Frequently, a thorough examination reveals nothing more than a healthy child with enlarged tonsils. As I always believe in giving the youngsters a break, I suggest deferring operation, and ask the mother to bring her child back again for a checkup before school starts again in September. I know that, during the summer, increased outdoor activity, with more of the body exposed to the ultraviolet rays of the sun, has a definite shrinking effect upon all lymphoid tissues, and the tonsils are by no means an exception. Therefore, when Nancy or Jimmy returns with Mother in the fall, I often am happy to find that examination shows complete freedom from tonsillitis and perfectly normal tonsils. Consequently, there is no need for removal of the tonsils, and I so inform the relieved parent.

From my own long experience with electrocoagulation of the tonsils and adenoids, I have come to the definite conclusion that it is not only the most adequate, but also the safest, technique for solving the tonsil problem. And I am pleased to say that I am not alone in this well-considered opinion. As far back as 1931, Dr. William Brady supported my view. Dr. Brady, as you very likely know, is a well-known medical writer whose syndicated column has been appearing in hundreds of newspapers all over the country for many years. He is also the author of the book: *An 80-Year-Old Doctor's Secrets of Positive Health.** An article by him published that year, said, in part:

> "I have never had my tonsils extirpated with diathermy or otherwise, but I'll tell the world that if mine had to come out, that's the way I'd like it. The old Spanish custom (ordinary surgical tonsillectomy) has always seemed to me a barbaric, crude, and most unsatisfactory procedure, even when performed by the most skilled specialists. Now that electrosurgery is established, acceptable and available wherever good doctors are to be found, I can only offer my sympathy and condolences to anyone who is compelled to submit to the snare or the guillotine."

* Prentice-Hall, Inc., Englewood Cliffs, N.J., 1961.

Please remember that this appraisal was written many years ago, and electrosurgery, quite new at that time, has come a long way since then. Today, my recommendation is that if you or any member of your family is troubled with tonsillitis, the family doctor should be consulted. He may decide that the trouble can be treated without consulting a specialist. On the other hand, if he feels that you should see an otolaryngologist, you can ask him to refer you to one who specializes in diathermic treatment of the tonsils, thus possibly avoiding their removal. Meanwhile, I rest my case on Dr. Brady's statement, which still holds good.

Doc Silvers says: "Despite all the advantages of civilized society, our senses of smell and taste have appreciably deteriorated. So keep your nose and throat clear and healthy, and you will relish your meals more, sense the delicate fragrance of the one you love, and appreciate the many other pleasant odors with which Nature abounds. You may even develop the keen sense of smell my dog Porgy enjoys."

Techniques for Safeguarding Your Sight

15 Of the five special senses, that of sight is most precious to us. It is also, in comparison, the most wonderful and intricately made. Today we have cameras which operate automatically, performing their functions at the touch of a button. But man has not constructed—nor ever will—a camera as perfect as the eye, which is provided with its own natural shutter, lens, and screen. It also adjusts automatically, accurately and instantly, is always in focus from about three feet to infinity, and unconsciously corrects itself for closer objects. In addition, our eyes "take pictures" in three-dimensional stereo, and in natural color besides.

how nature protects your eyes

In providing us with the extraordinary gift of sight, nature protects it well. The eye socket is surrounded by a bony case, between which is a thick layer of fibrous tissue that acts as a buffer against external forces. The eye also has a marvelous protective mechanism built into its anatomical structure, called the lacrimal glands, that are on each side of the eyes, lateral to them, and just below the temples. These are the tear-secreting glands, which are affected emotionally, and also by irritating chemicals and spices, as we learn when we peel an onion. Those in the acting profession use this bulb of a lily plant to make their dramatic expression more realistic. The eyeball and the inner surfaces of the lids are covered by a protective membrane (the conjunctiva), which is lubricated by the tears and a mucinous secretion from the tarsal glands buried in the lids. After flowing over the eye, they are drained into the nose by two small tubes (the naso-lachrymal ducts). Were it not for this continual cleansing and lubrication of the eyeball, the delicate membrane covering it would become dry and inflamed, and result in ulceration.

The tears contain lysozyme, a solution that prevents eye infection, which gets to the mouth by way of the ducts, there joining up with other protective and immunizing secretions from the mucous membrane of the mouth and throat. Those who are so fortunate as to have an abundance of these combined secretions will often check the development of that old-time misery, from which millions still suffer, known as the common cold, even when all about them are coming down with the sniffles. The immune factor has been isolated from the healthy nose and throat, and accounts for the lucky people who can be exposed to all kinds of nose and throat infections, and yet never succumb themselves.

don't waste beef steak on shiners

Man is an aggressive creature and, it seems, is always looking for a scrap. Despite nature's various protective devices, he will, upon occasion, get into a fist fight for some reason, or for no reason at all, and injure himself. The barbershops on the Bowery in New York, and in slum districts in other large cities, do a lucrative business in treating black eyes. Their practical therapy over many years is the application of a cold, wet slice of raw beef, after which the bruise is covered with flesh-colored greasepaint. I trust that my readers, if they *do* get into a scrap, will strike first and give the other fellow a black eye. However, if you unfortunately suffer this eye injury yourself, you can treat it without using raw beef, which, at today's prices, is an expensive therapy.

Home Rx for Black Eyes:

1) Add one heaping teaspoonful of powdered boric acid to one pint of hot water and stir.

2) Boil for three minutes.

3) Let cool and pour into a sterile bottle.

4) Keep from adding to this solution. Always pour out of the bottle and thus avoid contamination.

5) Using an eyecup, cleanse the eye with this solution.

6) Place a cold compress of the boric acid solution over the eye, renewing it as it gets warm, and continue for one hour.

7) Repeat these applications, one hour on and one hour off, until the redness and pain subside.

8) In 24 hours, if the condition is not relieved, see your doctor, who will probably prescribe an enzyme which, taken orally, will absorb the blood clot more rapidly.

While I do not expect that any of my women readers would get into a fracas resulting in a black eye, it might be noted, just in case, that this treatment is effective for the ladies as well as the men.

Doc Silvers says: "**The best protection against black eyes, to borrow a phrase from Theodore Roosevelt, is to 'speak softly and carry a big stick.'**"

Boric acid solution is a safe eyewash for home use, being anti-fungal and mildly antiseptic against the commoner eye infections. Good results are also obtained in the less serious infections of the conjunctiva (white) of the eyes with a mild (10%) protein silver solution (Argyrol). Dropped into the eye, it is highly efficient against pink eye, which is caused by a specific organism that not only turns the conjunctiva pink, but erupts a pus that makes the eyelids stick together during sleep.

Home Rx for Pink Eye:

1) Bathe the eye with boric acid solution to cleanse it of accumulated pus.

2) Drop two drops of the protein silver solution into the infected eye. The first drop washes away the mucus which covers the white of the eye; the second drop then acts without dilution.

3) Hold the head back and lift the upper lid so that the drops remain against the eyeball; keep this position for about one minute.

Two cautions about pink eye should be noted. It is highly contagious, the common agents being handkerchiefs and towels. Protein silver solution is deep brown and, if used for more than a week or two, enough silver may be deposited to stain the white of the eye a permanent blue, so use it sparingly and only for a brief period.

Emergency Treatment for Alkali and Acid Exposure

Should you accidentally get the fumes of ammonia or any other alkali into your eyes, immediately wash them out copiously with cold water. Then use the boric acid solution to neutralize the alkali. The same emergency treatment is indicated should you get lye into your eyes. It is important to act quickly to avoid permanent injury. Should inflammation and pain continue, see a doctor without delay.

When any acid gets into an eye, use the cold water emergency procedure just given. Follow with an alkali to neutralize the acid burn. Use bicarbonate or baking soda. Make up a solution by adding one heaping teaspoonful to one pint of sterile water. Use an eyecup for bathing the affected eye. Should the acid have been concentrated, your doctor will use a stronger neutralizing solution. We always try to neutralize the acid against the alkaline solution.

Removal of Foreign Particles

Any foreign substance, such as dust, grit, sand or dirt, that gets into an eye can usually be removed by washing it out with an eyecup of 0.9% clean salt water: one teaspoon salt to one pint of boiled, cold water. Follow this with boric acid solution for its mild sterilizing effect. Turning of the lid inside out, and removal by a cotton swab, dipped in the boric acid solution, is necessary when foreign matter clings to the mucus of the upper or lower lid. An imbedded substance must be removed aseptically by your doctor. Any abrasion which penetrates the cornea or conjunctiva of the eye requires professional attention. To avoid infection, your doctor will use one of the antibiotics.

Any inflammation of the eye may prove to be serious, so when in doubt, get medical advice. However, ordinary reddening of the eyes with allergic reactions is soon ruled out by past experience. Eyes may water and tears overflow, but you can get early relief by taking antihistaminic tablets, which are available from your druggist without prescription.

The Bugaboo of Eye Strain

One of the most common complaints doctors hear from their patients concerns what they generally term "eye strain." As a matter of fact, true eye strain is very rare. Bathing the eyes daily with so-called "colyrium for tired eyes" is worthless. Clearing the eyes in this way every day, as one brushes the teeth, is not only unnecessary but may prove harmful as it is practically impossible to keep the solution sterile for any length of time, and the polluted eyewash may then actually infect healthy eyes.

Doc Silvers says: **"Avoid interfering with unnecessary solutions, and let Mother Nature keep your eyes well lubricated and protected with her own healing and antiseptic fluids."**

The eye is a much tougher organ than most people realize. Reading or watching television for a protracted period may tire your eyes and cause them to smart and burn. However, this is easily explained when the function of blinking eyelids is understood. Each time you become intent, whether reading or viewing television, you retard the normal winking reflex action. On the under surface of each eyelid are tiny glands which secrete a lubricating fluid that anoints the white of your eyes, thus avoiding friction. A dry eye is a smarting and painful eye. You wink automatically and frequently when engaged in your daily tasks. It is only when you become engrossed at the movies, watching television, or intently reading for a prolonged time, that you do not wink sufficiently for proper lubrication. The solution to this common complaint is obviously simple, and you can perform it yourself quicker than a magician can pull a rabbit out of a hat. Just lubricate your conjunctiva with a few rapid winks. That's absolutely all there's to it. And on the same premise, should your eyes ever seem blurred and your vision indistinct, blink them a few times and note the immediate improvement. Blinking cleans away any interfering mucus, and thus clarifies your vision.

When one of these little glands under the eye lid becomes infected and inflamed, the duct is obstructed by the matter and a tumor (chalazion), which swells like a boil, develops. Hot compresses of boric acid will help bring it to a head. Often it may be checked if neomycin with triamcinolone, an ophthalmic ointment, is used soon enough. If, however, the swelling does not decrease after application of the ointment, it will be necessary for your doctor to release the pus by an incision.

Home Rx for Tired Eyes:

A gentle massage over the eyelids is often markedly relieving. Press the index and middle fingers lightly against the closed eyeball and massage from the lateral or outer border toward the nose with a circular motion. Just a few gentle strokes are all that's needed to provide you with many more hours of comfortable, tireless vision.

It is only when the eye muscles are brought into play for an extended period, or the light is poor, or your glasses are not functioning properly in focusing images on the retina, that you begin to feel your eye muscles tiring and, if you have a tendency to be hypersensitive, headache may ensue. This so-called "eye headache" is really an eye muscle pain due to overactivity, and corresponds to any other muscular strain.

Lighting with a minimum of glare is of prime importance for eye comfort. Always keep the source of light, as you would with a camera in taking a picture, in back of you. However, with modern light dispersion from a shaded lamp, you may read or write with the lamp in front of you, provided that the light is directed on the table and not into your eyes. In the early days of television, all room lighting had to be turned off. But with modern television receivers, the room can be softly lighted, and a shaded lamp, with not over a 15-watt bulb, should be placed on or above the set. In this way, with no sharp contrasts of light or darkness, you can watch television restfully if you turn your gaze away from the

picture occasionally, and remember to blink your eyes every now
and then.

Doc Silvers says: "Wink your eyes, keeping them clear and
sparkling, for as the poet said, they are 'the windows of the soul.'"

Simple Treatment for Styes

The common stye is an infection of the mucous membrane of
the eyelid. The medicalese for a stye is a hordeolum, which is
generally a staphylococcus infection that responds readily to one
of the antimicrobials like ophthalmic ointment of penicillin or neomycin combination. If you apply penicillin or one of the mycin
ointments soon enough, it will cause the swelling to recede before
it goes into the stage of pus formation. Should the inflammation
be marked and painful, one of the hydrocortisone synthetics like
neoaristocort ophthalmic ointment is indicated.

Always remember, as emphasized throughout this book, that
"an ounce of prevention is better than a pound of cure." In many
instances, we suffer needless pain because we do not know the
simple means of avoiding it. And, too, we often are infected because we do not observe ordinary hygienic care. Certain people
are particularly vulnerable to styes. Excessive use of the eyes, with
the resultant drying out of the mucosa at the border of the lids,
causes them to rub the itching area. Since the fingers are always
dirty, the resultant infection follows. The staphylococcus germ is
ubiquitous, being constantly present on unclean skin, and awaiting
the opportunity to invade the tissues.

Doc Silvers says: "Even amateur photographers know that they
must never touch the lens of a camera. Treat your sight with the
same meticulous care."

Professional Treatment of Eye Disorders

So far we have discussed emergency treatments and home
therapy for the common, simpler maladies of the eye, and prevention has been stressed. The eye is a very sensitive organ, one of

the most delicate in the body, and it is of extreme importance that your doctor, who may refer you to an ophthalmologist, be consulted whenever they are injured in any way. Therefore, before concluding this discussion of the eyes, I should like to review briefly the professional treatment of several familiar eye diseases. My principal purpose in doing so is to assure the reader that ophthalmology has become such a highly perfected science that there is no need for undue fear and trepidation when one of these malfunctions of the eye occurs. The eye doctor is a skilled medical technician who can literally—witness the eye banks—perform wonders today. So if one of these injuries should happen to you, do not be alarmed, but put your complete trust in him, just as you would in your spiritual advisor. You can rest assured that in his hands you will receive the very best of care, the trouble will be alleviated and, in many instances, completely cleared up.

Any injury of the eye in the region of the cornea (the colored portion, which includes the iris) requires expert medical attention. To prevent adhesions of the shutter mechanism, a 1% atropin solution is dropped into the affected eye. The one important contraindication to atropin (belladonna) is a hardened eyeball (glaucoma).

Glaucoma is due to faulty drainage of fluid from the anterior chamber of the eye, which is called aqueous humor, and protects the front of the lens. The watery fluid must have an outlet as it is secreted by the cells lining the sac. Normally, the fluid drains out via a channel known as the Canal of Schlemm. When this outlet is obstructed, the aqueous humor increases, and the eyeball gradually comes under greater pressure, resulting in excruciating pain. Hot compresses are indicated for relief until the doctor prescribes the essential constrictor of the iris, which is a 2% solution of pilocarpine. Permanent relief, and prevention of recurrence, is possible only by what is called an iridectomy. An incision is made through the iris, removing a portion, and so establishing drainage through the Canal of Schlemm. A myotic is often the prevention of damage to the eye which could cause blindness. By making the pupil smaller, the muscles of the iris release their pressure on the encircling canal for proper drainage. More of the aqueous humor can then escape from the anterior chamber, and the pressure drops.

Atropin, produced from the belladonna plant, is never used as it would increase the pressure within the anterior chamber by obstructing drainage, and thus lead to serious trouble. Belladonna, which means "beautiful woman," is so named because in ancient times women dropped a solution of the belladonna leaf into their eyes to enlarge the pupils, and thus increased their attractiveness. In the days of Cleopatra, this cosmetic application was quite the vogue. It is interesting to note, in this connection, that the belladonna plant is also known as the "deadly nightshade," which is a more appropriate name since it can be dangerous when used as a beauty aid. Today, fortunately, the lovely ladies do not drop belladonna into their eyes. Instead, they have turned to other exotic cosmetics, such as royal jelly (from the queen bee, no less), shark oil, and the extract of placenta. Ah, well!

Cataract is the gradual clouding of the lens of the eye. Normally, the light passes through a clear cornea, anterior chamber, lens, posterior chamber, and brings the image to rest on the retina in back of the eye. Any interference with the passage of this light through these media will affect the registration of the image. Clouding of the lens comes naturally with the aging process. However, complete obstruction to the light which passes through the cornea occurs only in a ripe or mature cataract. At that stage, the only recourse is to remove the opaque object, which is the lens. When it has been excised, there is no longer any obstruction to the light as it courses through to the retina. A substitute lens is then worn artificially as glasses, and the vision is brought back to as nearly normal as possible. Only in the elderly, where vascular involvement of the retina may be present, is there any difficulty with sight after a successful extraction of the opaque lens. The operation is now assisted by the enzymatic action of a substance which loosens up the attached fibers of the lens, thus considerably aiding the surgeon in removing the lens with a minimum of injury to the surrounding tissues.

The artificial substitution of lenses worn as ordinary spectacles does a perfect job, in almost all cases, and many people, who have had a cataract extraction comparatively early in life, are able to carry on at their normal tasks, with little inconvenience, for the rest of their days, thanks to the wonders of eye surgery.

Doc Silvers says: **"Guard your precious sight religiously and, meanwhile, contribute what you can for the help of the blind."**

Easy Ways to Protect Your Hearing

16 Before we can know how to take proper care of our hearing, we need to understand something about the way it functions. The ear consists of three parts, called, simply enough, the outer, middle, and inner ear. The outer ear comprises an appendage of cartilage and skin, the auricle or pinna, which collects the vibrations of sound and directs them into the ear canal, very much as a horn would. The drum or tympanum in the middle ear receives the vibrations as they enter. There they are amplified by a series of small ossicles (bones), three in number. The hammer or maleus is directly attached to the drum; adhering to the maleus is the anvil or incus; and attached to the incus is the third bone, called the stirrup or stapes. The stapes is attached to the window which separates the middle from the inner ear. It is the latter which lodges the vestibular canals and the organ of hearing, known as the cochlea.

The vibrations which reach the inner ear through the oval window are carried by a fluid that bathes the cochlea and the labyrinth of the vestibular apparatus, the organ of balance. Both of these delicate structures are imbedded in the meshwork of the mastoid bone, and each is covered on its inner surface with a receptive apparatus which, in turn, automatically transmits all impulses to a brain center. Any imbalance of the structure of either organ will result in a magnified disturbance which is telegraphed to the brain center specific for that function.

This capsule description is all we need know to appreciate that the ear, like the eye, is an intricate mechanism which requires attention and care. Nature protects our eyes and ears in ways that are

187

wondrous to contemplate. However, Nature, like the Lord, helps those who help themselves. Natural complaints can often be alleviated and cured by natural means. And so it is with the ears, as with every other part of the body. By protecting them, we frequently prevent the occurrence of illness and injury; and should they develop, we can, in many instances, check their progress by the proper use of simple remedies.

Treatment for Ear Wax

The outer ear is the only place in the entire body where a waxy substance, called sebum, is manufactured by special cells. The purpose of this bitter, acrid substance is to inhibit the entrance of insects into the delicate mechanism of the ear. Imagine what would happen to the ear drum if the wax were sweet like honey. We would be attacked by a swarm of bees every time we took a walk in the country, and we'd have to wear earmuffs to prevent our getting stung.

Impairment in hearing acuity is commonly due to wax in the external ear. Many people try to dig it out with the head of a match or the nail of the little finger. This is a dangerous practice. No foreign object should ever be inserted into the ear. All otologists constantly warn their patients. "Never stick anything into your ear except your elbow." However, there is a simple and safe way by which you may attempt to remove earwax.

Home Rx:

Before going to bed at night, fill a dropper full of peroxide and drop half into each ear. Then place cotton plugs in the ears to avoid leakage, and leave them in overnight. If the wax is not too hard and dry and impacted in the ear canal, the peroxide will soften it up and, when you remove the plugs in the morning, the wax will fall out by itself.

If this treatment does not afford relief, see an ear doctor before the condition worsens, for the longer you put it off, the more difficult, and perhaps painful, it will be to remove the wax. Ordinarily, if the accumulation of wax has not attached itself to the wall of the canal, the only treatment required is the use of an ear syringe filled with a warm 5% soda bicarbonate solution, which will wash it out. If this doesn't do the trick, there is a wax solvent (ceruminex) which, in the careful hands of the physician, will help soften and dislodge the wax, after which the syringe is used. When treatment has been inordinately delayed, the wax attaches itself to the skin of the external canal and, if removed by any means, will cause discomfort for a week or more. When the wax becomes attached, very much like a scab on the skin, bleeding will follow its removal if separation is impossible by the cerumen solvent. Removal of ear wax is not always easy, even for the experienced otolaryngologist who specializes in this field. However, if an accumulation of ear wax is promptly attended to, its removal is a simple and painless procedure. Therefore, may I emphasize again, in all matters which do not readily respond to home treatment, see your family doctor, or a specialist, if required, without delay. You will avoid needless pain, and save money, too.

treatments for motion sickness and migraine

You will remember that the labyrinth of the ear is the organ that controls balance, an extremely complicated and important function since, without it, we would all go stumbling around as if we were perennially intoxicated, which would never do.

A damaged or infected labyrinth leads to labyrinthitis (inflammation), and dizziness and faulty balance result. It may be objective, when the room and objects about you are apparently in motion; or subjective, when everything else is stationary, but you seem to be going around in a whirl. Practically everybody has experienced this dizzy feeling when subject to motion sickness. Car, train, sea, and plane sickness, so common in children and many adults, is due to a side-to-side motion which sends the labyrinthian fluid into wave-like, irritating impulses. The pitch of a ship from bow to stern is rarely upsetting. It is what is known to the mariner as the rolling of the vessel which makes even the most hardy a victim of seasickness. That is why you are apt to be upset by a crosscurrent trip, no matter how short, such as crossing the English Channel. It is the rolling of the ship, not necessarily rough seas, that determines the degree of whirling your labyrinthian canal is subject to.

Fortunately, as all experienced travelers know, there are many antimotion pills on the market today. Originally, sailors were given dramamine in 50 mg. doses to counteract seasickness. In this connection, it is interesting to note they discovered that the dramamine also provided relief from oncoming colds. It was this observation by those who sail the seven seas which brought on the use of the anti-histaminics as a preventive of the common cold. Another side effect, this one undesirable, is that dramamine in the required dosage has a soporific or sleep-inducing action. However, there are now improvements in medication which attempt to remove the resultant drowsiness of dramamine. Bonine and marezine are sedatives to the balancing mechanism of the inner ear. Taken a half-hour before starting a trip, whether by car, train, ship or plane, any of these antimotion drugs will protect you for many hours against dizziness, nausea, and subsequent vomiting.

Another affliction of the labyrinth is Meniere's Syndrome, a disease of the inner ear characterized by sudden deafness, which may be either acute or short-lived, or chronic and persistent, and requires the attention of a physician. He dilates the vessels of the labyrinth, thus helping to remove the fluid under pressure, by means of repeated doses of the vitamin Niacin in 100 mg. tablets. Niacin, unlike Niacinamide (both are otherwise alike), causes the patient to flush. The feeling of warmth is temporary, and usually lasts for just a few minutes. In the hypersensitive, half the dose is enough, and produces the essential dilatation which often so relaxes the patient that it will abort a migraine headache before it goes into the stages of dilatation.

Home Rx for Migraine:

Many a migraine headache can be prevented from developing into the excruciatingly painful stage experienced by its victims simply by taking vitamin Niacin in adequate dosage at the first sign of an attack. Migraine sufferers usually get ample warning: spots appear to obstruct vision (amblyopia) and flashes of light further complicate the picture; nausea comes early, and is later followed by headache and vomiting.

At the very first symptoms, even if they awaken you out of a sound sleep, immediately take 50 mg. of Niacin (formerly called Nicotinic Acid). If a flush ensues, the dose is sufficient to quickly dilate the constricted cerebral blood vessels. If you do not flush within ten minutes, take another tablet to produce the salutary flush or dilatation of the vessels of the skin. Presto—no migraine.

The latest theory on the cause of this type of headache is most interesting. The cerebral vessels first become constricted, and then greatly dilated. When you take Niacin during the early stage of constriction, you neutralize this stage, and so prevent the excessive dilatation which normally would follow, and which is the cause of the characteristic splitting headache, always on one side of the head.

Doc Silvers says: "Avoid the reaction, a la Isaac Newton. Old Isaac knew what he was talking about when he promulgated the third law of motion: 'Every action has an equal and opposite (potent) reaction.'"

How to Handle "Athlete's Foot" of the Ear

The commonest disease of the canal of the ear, called Otitis Externa, is caused by a fungus or large germ in the skin of the canal, and requires professional treatment. If a fungus is present, it is called Otomycosis. The fungi like it dark, moist, and warm, and an alkaline medium, which is why they thrive between the toes, arms, legs, and in the outer ear. Antifungal preparations are indicated, one of the most effective being a mixture of equal parts of vinegar and ethyl alcohol. When the inflammation is so disturbing that life becomes difficult, corticotropic hormone in the form of an ointment of triamcinolone with neomycin is applied by the doctor. This alleviates the itching and extreme discomfort of the infested skin, and so hastens healing.

Treatment of Earache

Earache may be due to trouble inside or outside the ear. The commonest form of pain in the ear comes with an infection of the nose and throat. Several days after a head cold, sudden pain in an ear usually means that an infection has spread to the inner ear via the (Eustachian) tube from the back of the nose. Only your doctor can determine the extent of infection and damage to the eardrum.

Home Rx:

For emergency treatment, should it occur in the middle of the night as it commonly does with children, a few drops of pure glycerine, slightly warmed by holding the bottle in the hand, may be dropped into the ear. Or fill the ear canal with about four drops of 1% phenol in glycerine for quicker relief of pain. Your druggist has many forms of glycerine ear drops, some containing a sulpha drug along with a local anesthetic, for the treatment of excruciating pain. The glycerine has a hygroscopic (condensing) action which helps absorb the excess fluid in the middle ear, relieving the pressure against the drum membrane, hence reducing the swelling and pain. Be sure that the dropper does not touch the skin of the outer ear as you apply the drops to the side wall of the external canal. No water should be used to cleanse the dropper as it would dilute the pure glycerine.

Play Safe When Swimming

The best therapy there is for diseases of the internal ear—as with many other ailments, as this book demonstrates—is *prevention*.

During the summer months, when we go on vacation, swimming is one of the our most healthful and delightful sports. Be it the brine of the sea, or the fresh water of an upland lake, it is a beneficial and refreshing form of exercise. However, before swimming, we should always take the few simple precautions required to protect our ears from infection.

Before entering the water, pack your ears with a little molded lamb's wool. If you are a beginner at diving or jumping, close your nostrils with a pair of rubber nose clips. This is imperative for those who have perforated eardrums and swim in water which may be polluted.

The eardrum is normally impervious to water, and the middle or inner ear cannot be infected by way of an external approach. All inner ear infections start for the first time via the nose and throat. Infection is begun by the passage of water through the openings behind the soft palate (uvula) to the Eustachian Canals, which go directly to the middle ear and balance the pressure on the eardrums. The entrances to these canals are normally open. If there is an obstruction to the passageway, the drums are damaged on a change of pressure, such as when mountain climbing or flying in a plane. The external pressure at sea level is about fifteen pounds per square inch. Any change from this pressure must be equally distributed to both sides of the eardrums. If this does not occur, the drums can no longer vibrate freely, and hearing is impaired. It then becomes necessary to have a doctor dilate the Eustachian Tubes by air pressure to keep them open. If this is not done soon following Eustachian Tube Catarrh, the victim will be left with permanently impaired hearing.

The commonest ear ailment during the bathing season is swimmer's ear. Infection while swimming, diving, or fetching under water, follows a head cold (nasopharyngitis). The water, via the nose, carries the infection into the tubes leading to the middle ear. Otitis Media Catarrhalis Acuta—which is a mouthful, or perhaps I should say an earful—is medicalese for an infected and painful middle ear in its early stages. Fortunately, we no longer fear the dreaded mastoid complication of former days. The indicated antimicrobials are a blessing, and only very rarely does the condition become acute, or develop into a permanently discharging ear, as of yore. Now we can usually nip the infection in the bud and save the hearing, whereas before the wonder drugs arrived, we commonly saw a complicating mastoiditis develop within a few weeks after an ear became chronically involved. Today, mastoiditis has disappeared, along with the horse and buggy, and we do not even have cases for demonstration to medical students in their operative training in the field of otolaryngology, the study of ear, nose and throat diseases. Although medicine still has a good way to go, it has already come a long way, and we all have much to be thankful for.

By the simple procedure of preventing polluted water from entering the middle ear, either via the perforated eardrum of an old acute infection, or via the nose while plunging, diving or jumping into the water, literally tens of thousands of cases of ear infection may be avoided each year. Remember, water can only get to your middle ear through a perforated drum, or be washed into it forcefully through the nose, via the Eustachian Tube, while dunking in the water. So all the simple protection you need is lamb's wool to protect a perforated drum and act as ear stopples, and rubber nose clips to keep your nostrils closed when plunging into the water. Then you'll always be playing safe while swimming.

How to Feel Young, Stay Young and Live Longer

17 Many home remedies and preventions have been given throughout this book for the promotion of health and longevity. They are all simple and they are all effective. By using them as needed and directed, you can be healthier and add years of active, happy life to your statistical span.

To help you achieve this desirable goal, your family doctor, and the specialists he consults, are always available to you. In addition, your pharmacist compounds your prescriptions carefully and accurately. With this team rooting for you, the future is brighter than ever before. Preventive medicine today is making great strides in avoiding the ills common to mankind. Medical science has been eminently successful in the fight against tuberculosis, polio, venereal disease, among many other ailments, and will soon conquer cancer. This era is called the Space Age, the Electronic Age, and the Age of Automation. It might also well be called the Age of Medical Discovery.

Life expectancy at birth has doubled within the past century. But—and note this well—man does not presently live any longer than his ancestors did. The statistical increase of life expectancy is principally due to the fact that many more babies survive because most deliveries are now made in hospitals, where hygienic conditions are paramount. Up until recent years, the emphasis was on keeping the newborn alive, and that aim, of course, still continues. But today, with a constantly increasing older population, geriatrics, the branch of medical science dealing with the problems and diseases of aging, is receiving ever greater attention, and already is keeping millions of older folk alive, who would have died much earlier a generation or two ago.

This shift in medical research from the early to the later years of life is of immense importance to all of us. It means that you and I can remain healthier, more active, and add more years to our lives. According to the Bible, Moses lived to the ripe old age of 120; Noah was around for 950 years; and Jared for 962. Methuselah beat them all by living into his 969th year. Today scholars question how long these years might have been. If it assumed that they equaled our seasons—approximately three months, that is—then Moses died at 30 years of age, while Methuselah didn't attend his own funeral until he was over 242 years old. Perhaps some historian flunked in mathematics, or maybe these are just typographical errors. We'd best leave that puzzler to the biblical scholars. The important point to us in the twentieth century is that every child born today, receiving the immense advantage of modern medicine's preventive inoculations, should, barring physical accident, live appreciably longer than his grandparents. And at the other end of life's span, it is much easier for us adults to live up to the century mark.

How Young Are You?

If you are to live all your years to the hilt, of especial significance is your attitude toward life itself. The fundamental fault is that we measure a man's age chronologically, not taking into consideration that, however old he may be, he can still be young at heart. This ancient method is outdated and should be discarded forthwith. I am sure that some bright young psychologist can devise a more representative means of measurement which would incorporate a man's mental and emotional age on a psychological scale of values, irrespective of when he was born. Then women, when asked their age in registering to vote, wouldn't have to smirk and say, "Over 21." Instead, they could proudly declare, "I'm a P-25," or whatever their psychological rating, even if they were ninety. So forget your calendar age and concentrate on having a youthful attitude toward life.

Doc Silvers says: "Young girls may be pretty; but it takes years of understanding and compassion, experience and wisdom, friendliness and love, to make a woman truly beautiful."

How to Live Longer

Scores of simple home remedies have been prescribed in these pages for the various ailments of man and woman. It has been stated, you will remember, that many common illnesses can be prevented, and others may be aborted or cured by following the fundamental principles of physical medicine. All of these naturally contribute—in addition to their immediate beneficial effect—to better health and longer life. But medication in itself is not the whole story. Doctors and specialists can help you only so much; the rest is your own responsibility. And you have a great advantage in this respect for you are the only living creature on the face of the earth who, instead of acting by instinct, can reason, thereby determining, in large measure, your own destiny. So in this final chapter, let us put aside prescriptions, preventives, and potions, and concentrate upon the things in everyday life which we can control by our own will. Kahlil Gibran, the mystical Syrian poet, emphasized how important they are. "Your daily life," he wrote, "is your temple and religion." If we follow this philosophy, we can do much to extend our years, and make them richer and more enjoyable.

Vascular diseases are our most common ailments, and result, by far, in the greatest number of fatalities. A major contributing factor is high blood pressure. People discuss their diastolic and systolic pressures as casually as farmers talk about the weather. "How's your blood pressure today?" is a familiar greeting among friends. We Americans become tense and tied up in knots under the constant pressure of getting ahead, earning more money, and keeping up with the Smiths as well as the Joneses. Relaxing home remedies were given earlier. However, there is more that we can do to lead well-regulated lives, thus reducing our tensions and our blood pressure, as well.

Have a Good Belly Laugh

Just as belly breathing benefits the constitution generally, so does the belly laugh. The best medicine for the tensions under which we live is a good sense of humor. It is an effective antidote for the blues. A pleasing smile and a happy heart can work wonders for all of us. Don't just laugh at the other fellow; laugh at yourself upon occasion and it will do much for your morale. Hearty laughter helps to control the harmful emotions of anger, hate, and jealousy. It holds your blood pressure down, keeps you from worrying needlessly, and makes a stroke much less likely. Though it may seem unladylike, I advocate the belly laugh for women, too.

Take Frequent Vacations

I recommend, you will remember, eating as often each day as you wish, as much as six times, if you like. As long as you stay within your daily caloric requirement, it is much better, especially as you get older, to eat a little at a time, rather than overwork your heart in digesting large meals. Along the same line, I also advise several vacations annually instead of just one. I know a couple who go away four times a year, each trip consisting of a long weekend from Thursday to Monday inclusive. They live in New York City and, what with the speed of jet travel, are able to weekend in the Midwest, the South, Canada, Bermuda, and the Bahamas. And yet these four short trips keep them away from their work only twelve business days a year.

Quietude and recreation are both essential to a well-rounded life. Get away from the routine of the daily task periodically, even if for just a little while. Occasional brief vacations will do more toward refreshing and revitalizing you than a long one that might overtax you if you indulge in active recreation to which you are unaccustomed, or may bore you to death if you just loll around.

Doc Silvers says: "Just as several small sectors of strawberry shortcake are more pleasurable than one large slab that may make

you ill, so several short vacations are more enjoyable than a long one which may exhaust you."

don't argue unnecessarily

The home atmosphere is a most important factor in the enjoyment and prolongation of life. Every tenet of good health revolves around the relationship of husband and wife. If peace does not reign in the home, food cannot be properly digested. The enzymes and juices so essential to normal digestion are dried up in the heat of argument, especially if it occurs at mealtime. Most of the gastrointestinal complaints after partaking of good food are due to mental, rather than physical, disturbances.

Your home is your *sanctum sanctorum*, and meals should be an integral part of that peaceful privacy. Make it an incontrovertible rule never to discuss anything controversial while at the dining table. If you must argue, wait for an hour after a meal, and then put it off for another hour, if at all possible.

Doc Silvers says: "The best time for an argument is the day after tomorrow."

It is the simple and the common which affect us from hour to hour. Unnoticed, our blood pressure rises from repetition of the most trivial occurrences. I well remember the simple philosophy expounded by a Monsignor I treated some years ago. We had been discussing the common problem of how a tired, tense husband is greeted when he comes home after a hard day's work, and I voiced the opinion that an understanding wife would respond to his mood by making everything as agreeable and comfortable as possible. The elderly Monsignor looked up at me from deep thought and said, "God made woman to be the pincushion of man." Certainly the wise wife accepts these pinpricks as part of her obligation in making their home life pleasant. I have seen many a wholesome and nutritious meal lead to heartburn and indigestion needlessly occasioned by a few injudicious remarks made by either spouse.

And yet it is easy to avoid these useless episodes and their consequences just by a little give and take on both sides.

Doc Silvers says: "When you're eating, don't argue; if you
argue, don't eat."

how to achieve harmonious
sexual intimacy in marriage

In this morning's paper, as I write, I read an account of a con-
ference at the University of California Medical Center on the subject, "Man and Civilization; The Family's Search for Survival."
One of the speakers was Dr. Lester A. Kirkendall, professor of
family life at Oregon State University, who declared that attacks
should be made upon specific sexual taboos in the family. He urged
educational programs to "deal realistically with the foundation of
sexual morality" and "rid ourselves of the common paralyzing fear
of sex, which leaves us both tongue-tied and blind to reality."

Cooperative sexual congress is a most important factor in har-
monious family life. In the scores of surveys on marital problems
which I have seen over the years, misunderstanding in matters
sexual has invariably been given as the most prevalent, financial
running a poor second. Certain it is that sexual release is man's most
continually effective biological means of enjoyment and relaxation.
Man's sexual urge is, in fact, so strong that, as newspaper headlines
regularly confirm, it can lead to crimes of violence, even murder.

It is difficult for a woman to understand and appreciate the over-
whelming power of man's biological desire. There are two precise
reasons for this lack of knowledge so necessary to happiness in
married life. The natural one is that a woman's passions are much
less easily aroused and, consequently, it takes her appreciably longer
to reach a climax. The other comes from the fact that our so-called
"modern society" still will not permit educators to teach the fun-
damentals of a sane sex life in our schools. In this connection, note
that providing sex education in universities, as some few do, is too
late. It must be given in public schools at the time when youngsters
are going through the major biological changes occurring during

puberty. Thus, instead of being frustrated, and often frightened, they will understand and be prepared to adjust to them intelligently.

The husband whose sexual urges have been properly fitted into the pattern of married life with the willing cooperation of his wife is a far more contented, and even saner, man than one whose biological desires are subject to the whims and fancies of unpredictable chance.

We know that a long and enjoyable life depends upon health, nutrition, exercise, relaxation, and rest. Sexual compatibility plays a major role in providing pleasure, relaxation, untroubled sleep, and deep contentment. It is, therefore, a prime factor in insuring emotional and mental stability, thus substantially contributing to general good health and a fuller, longer life.

Since man is demanding, woman should be understanding. And it is not nearly as difficult as she may think. Like all members of my profession, I have in my long practice had innumerable opportunities to observe the intimate problems which all too frequently arise in married life. And I have several suggestions to make which, to my best knowledge, have not been advanced before, to those loving couples who may suspect that their marital relationship is perhaps not all it can be.

helping women over their difficult days

The large majority of married women keep a calendar record of their menses for the purpose of checking regularity and the possibility of conception. Because of society's hypocritical attitude toward sex, they secrete this important family record, thinking it shameful, and hide it from their husband's eyes. However, he should be able to consult this calendar at any time, thus enabling him to adjust his desires to the periodicity of the menses. Nothing disturbs a husband more than to find that his mounting passion must be kept in leash until the menstrual flow has ceased. Therefore, in having free access to this record, and frankly discussing it, instead of coitus on a haphazard basis, definite arrangements can be agreed upon.

The Secret of Compatibility

I have emphasized that health and happiness in daily life are founded upon regularity and reasonableness in all things. This definitely includes the sexual relationship. Dr. Kirkendall, previously quoted, said, "One taboo prohibits adults from recognizing themselves as sexual beings unless it is done with frivolity, or in a spirit of braggadocio." The enjoyment of sensual congress is not lessened by planning; rather, it is heightened by pleasurable anticipation. Every fundamental factor in family life should be arranged and, in the same way, couples should keep on having dates after marriage, as they did before. They are, in fact, more important then because during the honeymoon the wonders and delights of biological responses can be intimately explored. The couple who plan "love dates" throughout marriage, just as they arrange the other basic factors, will be blessed with all the many beneficences of a well-ordered life. Misunderstandings and arguments, and the consequent tensions and physical upsets, will be infrequent, and such "lovers' quarrels" quickly overcome through mutual understanding and deep-seated affection. As a result, their marriage, barring accident, will be a long and happy one because they are relaxed and content.

Doc Silvers says: "In the privacy of marriage, there is nothing shameful about sex unless thinking makes it so."

How Not to Retire

In the continuing study of geriatrics, it is being found that retirement *per se* is often psychologically undesirable. When asked about it, Bernard Baruch said, "I do not believe in discarding human beings." No one should retire from life until life retires from him. Nicholas Murray Butler, the late educator, who was president of Columbia University for over forty years, once observed that the tombstone of a great many people should read, "Died at thirty; buried at sixty." Given normal health, there is no reason why you should contemplate retirement. Many a man has looked forward to it with pleasurable anticipation, and died soon after on finding that he no longer had anything to live for. After all, the universal wish for long life is predicated upon the human desire to add to one's active, enjoyable years.

If you are doing a good job at your daily task, have a feeling of pride in your accomplishments, and receive the sincere praise of those about you, do not retire so long as your health and legal status permit you to carry on. It is all wrong to make retirement mandatory at sixty-five, or any other age, for that matter. Many statistical surveys prove that our senior citizens are more productive, have greater skill in their jobs, accomplish more with less effort, and have a better absentee record, than workers half their age. As a result, unjustified prejudice against older people is gradually being overcome.

Enlarge Your Interests

Don't wait until the retirement age to find something to do with your time afterwards. Engage in some extracurricular interest now so that you can continue to be active when you are no longer engaged in your regular vocation. Keeping occupied and enjoying it is the secret of the inner urge for accomplishment. We are all driven by two primary forces. The *vis a tergo*, or force from within, previously mentioned, directs our energies in spite of ourselves, leading us to do things we thought were impossible of attainment. It is that which has made leaders of men; it is that which makes us "do or die." The other great force is the *vis a fronte*, or force from without, which promotes our ambition and drives us to accomplishment. It is that which we do gratis just for the gratification it brings us. It is evidenced in communal and social work, and other voluntary endeavors.

How to Live Longer

When you are willing and eager to do something for nothing, you are engaged in a pleasurable pursuit. In directing this energy toward a cause really worth your while, you will be doubly blessed: the gratification you get from personal accomplishment, and the plaudits you receive from those who appreciate a good job well done. It is this stimulus which you will need after your days of gainful employment are over. So plan ahead now.

If you wish to live long, you have a much better chance to do so today. Growth goes with knowledge. If you wish to continue to grow, you will never give up learning. The man who gradually loses interest in life and the world about him is slowly committing suicide. As the homely saying has it, "he is dead but doesn't know enough to lie down."

The zest for living is most essential to long life. There are many examples today—you know them as well as I—of individuals who never stop adding to their knowledge, even into their eighties and beyond. There will be greater numbers in the years to come who will remain active, productive, and still interested in life even as centenarians. He who would live long must have a pronounced desire to do so.

Having conquered the diseases of childhood, we shall eventually overcome those of premature senility. One need not be an oracle to predict with conviction that in future generations—perhaps your children; certainly your grandchildren—it will be common to observe men and women a hundred years old who are engaged in various pleasurable pursuits; an avocation, an art, a hobby, playing various games, dancing and singing with joy in their hearts.

I recently saw a delightful little porcelain figure of the Japanese concept of Father Time. There was a smile on his lips and a twinkle in his eyes. He wore a long, flowing, white beard and, except for the oriental costume covering his roly-poly body, he looked just like our Santa Claus.

It is perfectly natural to grow old. You start aging the moment after conception. Constant replacement of your body cells throughout the years keeps you from the process of degeneration. If you supply your bodily needs with wholesome, nutritious food, and observe regularity in your work, recreation, exercise, and rest, you can avoid the process of deterioration in large measure. Use the sound medical precepts given in this book as your guide. Then you will be pleasurably active to a hundred and older, and your later days will be years of moderate and gradual recession, rounding out a long, vigorous, healthful, useful, and enjoyable existence.

Doc Silvers says: "Don't visualize death as a black-robed ghoul with a scythe. Instead think of Mother Nature, who toiled millions of years to fashion the wonder of man, and is perfectly willing to patiently await your return to her bosom. So live life, love life, and bide your time."

Index

A

Acidity, 123, 169
Acidophilus milk, 116
Acne, 55, 149
Addictions, drug, 131-133
Adenoids, 174
Aging, 148-150, 195-205
Air bathing, 71-73
Air conditioning, 150
Alcoholic drinks, cold, 122
Alcoholism, 132-133, 155
Alkaline baths, 142
Allergies:
  eyes, 181
  foods, 172
  hay fever, 158
  milk, 92
  poison ivy, 143-144
  pollens, 158
Almond oil, 149
Alpha keri, 60
Amblyopia, 191
American Medical Association, 155
Ammonia, aromatic spirits of, 71
*An 80-year-Old Doctor's Secrets of
  Positive Health*, 174
Angstrom Units, 38-39
Antifungal preparations, 191
Antihistaminics, 143, 158, 172, 181, 190
Antimotion pills, 190
Anxiety, effect on digestion, 100
Apples, pectin in, 99
Aqueous humor, of eyes, 184-185
Arguments, and health, 199
Argyrol, 179, 180
Artificial sunlight, benefits of, 53-54
  see also Light therapy; Sunlamps;
  Ultraviolet radiation
Asiatic influenza, 162

Aspirin, 164, 168
Asthma, bronchial, 62
Atherosclerosis, 92
"Athlete's ear," 145
"Athletes foot," of skin, 144-145
Atropin, 184, 185
Australia, Kenny method in, 26
Aveeno Oilated, 149-150
Aveeno Soap Cake, 148, 150

B

Back arch exercise, 85
Balance, sense of, 189-190
Baldness, 146-148
Balneotherapy (spa bathing), at home,
  60-61
Baruch, Bernard, 148, 202
Basal metabolism, 65
Basic Daily Dietary, 107-108
Basic Daily Dietary (chart), 91
Baths, 49-56, 57-67, 135-136, 142, 149-
  150 *see also* Water therapy
Belladonna, 184, 185
Belly breathing, 78-80
Bicycle riding exercise, 82-83
Bile stoppage, in liver, 80
Bioflavonoids, 94 *see also* Vitamins
Biomydrin, 157
Bladder irritations, 62
Bladder stones, 28
Blood circulation *see* Circulation
Blood clots, 92
Blood pressure, 27, 62, 80, 197, 198, 199
Blood vessel diseases, 92, 112 *see also*
  Circulation; Heart diseases
Body, heat regulatory powers of, 64
Body heat, 73-74
Boils, 55, 151-152
Bone fractures, 35, 46

207

Bonine, 190
Borated talcum, 145
Boric acid solutions, 178-179, 180
Brady, Dr. William, 174-175
Bread, 93-94
Breast milk, 95
Breathing, 78-80
Breathing, shortness after exercise, 84
Brewer's yeast, 92
Bronchitis, chronic, 62
Brophy, John, 140
Burns, 145-146
Burns, Robert, 16
Butler, Nicholas Murray, 202
Butter fat, 116, 117
Butter substitutes, 116
Buttermilk, 101

C

Caffeine, 121
Calamine solution, phenolated, 153
Calcium, 54-55
California, University of, 200
Calorie Allowances (table), 105, 107
Calories, daily consumption, 105-107
Camphor, 164
Canal of Schlemm, 184
Canker sores, 171-172
Carbohydrates, in diet, 113
Casals, Pablo, 148
Cataracts, 185-186
Catarrhal infections see Colds
Cerebral vascular diseases, 92
Ceruminex, 189
Chalazion, 182
Cheyn, George, 104
Cholesterol, 118
Churchill, Winston, 76
Cigarette smoking see Smoking
Circulation, blood, 28, 32, 45, 80, 110, 164
Citrus fruits, 94
Climatotherapy, 64-65, 73-74
Cod liver oil, 56
Coffee, 121, 135
Cold alcoholic drinks, 122
Cold compresses, for inflammation, 31-32
Cold cream, 141-142, 149
Cold drinks vs. hot, 122
Cold and heat, use of, 31-35
Cold hypertonic salt solutions, for sinus headaches, 157
Cold water, for burns, 145-146
Cold water bathing, safety rules, 66-67
Cold water therapy, 58-59

Colds:
    avoidance, 159-160
    blowing of nose, 164-165
    contagiousness, 160
    and eyes, 178
    facts concerning, 160
    fever, 164
    foot bath, hot mustard, 163
    home prescriptions, 163-164
    hot drinks, 163, 164
    immunization against influenza, 162
    list of preventive measures, 161-162
    nasal sprays, 164
    prevention, 155-156, 161-162
    quinine medication, 163
    sweating, 163
    viruses, 160
Colloidal emollient baths, 149-150
Colon, putrefactive bacteria in, 116-117
Common cold see Colds
Compatibility, in sex, 202
Compresses:
    cold, 31-32, 34-35, 157
    effective use of, 34-35
    hot, 26, 33-34, 152, 182, 184
Conjunctiva, 40, 177-178
Constipation, 46, 98-101, 150-151
Cooked food vs. raw, 94-96
Cornea, 40
Coronary artery diseases, 92, 112
Corticotropic hormone, 191
Cosmetics, 139-142, 185
Cottage cheese, 92
Cough medicines, 167-169
Cowper, William, 92
Cowpox, 27
Cramps, muscle, 43-44
Crime, and drug addiction, 131
Curare, 27

D

Dark glasses, 41
Deadly nightshade, 185 see also Bella·donna
Delirium tremens, 132-133
Dermatophytosis, 144-145
Dermis, 150 see also Skin
Desquamation, 39
Diaphragm, 79-80
Diaphragmatic breathing, 78-80
Diarrhea, 99
Diathermocryptectomies, 173
Diet (See also Reducing):
    anxiety, 100
    apples, 99

Diet (*cont.*)
  Basic Daily Dietary (chart), 91
  bread, 93-94
  breast milk, 95
  buttermilk, 101
  citrus fruits, 94
  constipation, 46, 98-101, 150-151
  cottage cheese, 92
  daily vitamin requirements, 91
  eggs, 112
  "enriched" bread, 94
  fats, 112, 116, 117, 118
  fish, 111, 112
  flour, 93-94
  insecticides in food, 93
  iron, 99
  lecithin, 92
  malt soup extract, 101
  meal times, 96-98
  meat, 95-96, 112, 117
  milk, 92, 95, 99, 116-117
  natural foods, 92
  natural laxatives, 98-101
  oils *see* Oils
  overeating, 96, 97
  pasteurized milk, 95
  potatoes, 94
  poultry, 112
  raw *vs.* cooked foods, 94-96
  restaurants, 97-98
  roughage, 99
  servings, 97
  soya beans, 92
  trichinosis, 95-96
  veal, 112
  vitamins *see* Vitamins
  wheat germ, 92
Digestion, effect of anxiety on, 100
Digitalis, 27
Discomfort Index, 65-66
Diverticulitis, 99
Dramamine, 190
Dropsy, 27
Drowning, 66-67
Drug addictions, 131-133
Drugs, expenditures for, 98
Dry heat, 42
Duodenal ulcers, 123

E

Ears:
  anatomy, 187
  antimotion pills, 190
  "athlete's foot" of, 191
  earache, 192

Ears (*cont.*)
  eardrum, 193
  Eustachian Tube Catarrh, 193
  fungi diseases, 191
  glycerine ear drops, 192
  infections, 159, 165, 193
  inner-ear infections, 193
  labyrinthian canal, 189-190
  labyrinthitis, 189
  massage, 182
  mastoiditis, 193-194
  Meniere's Syndrome, 190
  middle-ear diseases, 165
  motion sickness, 189-190
  Otitis Externa, 191
  Otitis Media Catarrhalis Acuta, 193
  otomycosis, 191
  sebum, 188-189
  sense of balance, 189-190
  swimming, 192-194
  wax, 188-189
Eating habits, 120-121 *see also* Diet;
    Reducing
Edema, 27
Effleurage, 44-45 *see also* Massage
Egg white, for skin injuries, 153
Eggs, in diet, 112
Elbow push exercise, 85
Elbow stretch exercise, 84
Electrocoagulation, 173, 174
Electrosurgery, 173, 174-175
Elevated scissors exercise, 86
Elizabeth I, queen of England, 27
England, 27
Enzymes:
  eye injuries, 179
  eye operations, 185
  inflammations, 35
  meat processing, 117
Epidermis, 150 *see also* Skin
Ergosterol, 38, 54
Erythema, 39-40
Eskimos, 112, 156
Essay on Man, 139
Estivin, 158
Estrogen, 92
Eustachian Canals, 193
Eustachian Tube Catarrh, 193
Eustachian tubes, 159, 160, 192, 193, 194
Exercises, 77-89
  back arch, 85
  belly breathing, 78-80
  bicycle riding, 82-83
  breathing, 78-80
  diaphragmatic breathing, 78-80
  elbow push, 85

Exercises (*cont.*)
elbow stretch, 84
elevated scissors, 86
extended sit-up, 84
gravity-eliminated, 87
hip twisting, 83
isometrics, 87-88
isotonics, 87
knee flexing, 82
knee push, 85
leg lift, 85
lying down, 81-87
progress report, 86
and recreation, 88-89
and reducing, 85
resistance exercises, 87-88
right angle, 87
scissors, 86
shortness of breath after, 84
shoulder curling, 82
after showers, 81
sit-up, 84
stretch over, 83
swimming, 80-81
Extended sit-up exercise, 84
Extremes, 39
Exudates, 45
Eyeglasses, dark, 41
Eyes:
acid exposure, 180
alkali exposure, 180
allergic reactions, 181
ammonia exposure, 180
aqueous humor, 184-185
"black eyes," 178-179
blinking, 181-182
Canal of Schlemm, 184
cataracts, 185-186
chalazion, 182
colds, 178
"colyrium for tired eyes," 181
conjunctiva, 177-178
cosmetics, 185
dark glasses, 41
enzymes for injuries, 179
"eye headache," 182
eyewashes, 181
foreign particles, 180-181
glaucoma, 184-185
immunizing secretions, 178
infections, 179, 182, 183
inflammations, 180-181
lacrimal glands, 177
light and glare, 182
and light therapy, 37
lye exposure, 180

Eyes (*cont.*)
lysozyme, 178
naso-lachrymal ducts, 178
natural protection, 177-178
pink eye, 179-180
professional treatment of disorders, 183-186
reading, 181
staphylococcus infections, 183
strain, 181-182
styes, 183
sunburn of, 40-41
tarsal glands, 178
tears, 177-178
television, 181
winking reflex, 181

F

Fats, polyunsaturated, 112, 116, 117, 118
Fever, 32, 164
Fish, Composition of (table), 111
Fish, in diet, 111
Fish oils, 56, 112
Flaxseed poultice, 61
Florida, 74, 75
Flour, 93-94
Foods, natural, 92 *see also* Diet
Foods, raw *vs.* cooked, 94-96
Foot baths, hot, 61-62, 163
Fosdick, Harry Emerson, 148
Foxglove (digitalis), 27
Fractures, 35, 46
Franklin, Benjamin, 120, 148
Friction, in massage, 46-47
Fungus infections, 55, 144-145, 191
Furunculosis, 55

G

Gall bladder trouble, 121, 122
Gentian violet, 171
Geriatrics, 149, 195, 205
Germany, trichinosis in, 96
Gibran, Kahlil, 197
Glaucoma, 184-185
Glycerine ear drops, 192
Glycogen, 132
Gravity-eliminated exercises, 87
Green soap, tincture of, 153
Guaiacol, 168

H

Habit *vs.* addiction, 132-133
Habits, formation of, 120-121

Hair, baldness, 146-148
Halitosis, 171
Harvard School of Public Health, 115
Hats, and baldness, 147
Hay fever, 158 *see also* Allergies; Nose
Headaches, migraine, 190-191
Headaches, from sinus infections, 34
  157-158
Hearing *see* Ears
Heart diseases, 27, 62, 92, 97, 110, 118,
  169
Heartburn, 123
Heat:
  and blood circulation, 28
  of body, 73-74
  and cold, use of, 31-35
  dry, 42
  infrared light therapy, 42
  regulation by body, 64
  relief from, 71
  strokes, 39
Heliotherapy, 69-76 *see also* Light
  therapy
High blood pressure *see* Blood pressure
Hip twisting exercise, 83
Hippocrates, 17
Histamine, 38, 39
Hives, 144
Holmes, John Haynes, 148
Home atmosphere, 199
Home massage *see* Massage
Honey, 124-125
Hordeolum, 183
Hot compresses:
  for eyes, 182, 184
  for pimples, 152
  in polio treatment, 26
  salt solutions in, 33-34
Hot drinks, 121-123
  for common cold, 163, 164
  for insomnia, 135
  vs. cold drinks, 122
Hot foot baths, 61-62, 163
Hot hypertonic salt solution, 34
Hot packs, for pain, 61
Hot salt solutions, for throat, 170
Hot water therapy, 59-61
The Human Face, 140
Humor, sense of, 198
Husbands and wives, 199-202
Hydrochloric acid, in removal of in-
  secticides in food, 93
Hydrocortisone ointments, 183
Hydrotherapy, 57-67
Hypertonic baths, 142
Hypertonic salt solutions, 33-34

Hypnotic drugs, 133
Hypochondria, 129

I

Ichthyosis, 142
Infant mortality, U.S., 95
Infantile paralysis, 25-28
Infectious gingivitis, 170-171
Inflammations:
  cold compresses, 31-32
  enzymes, 35
  hot compresses, 33-34
Inflammatory matter (exudates), 45
Influenza, immunization against, 162
Infrared light therapy, 42
Insect bites, relief from, 70-71
Insecticides, in food, 93
Insomnia, 62, 80, 129-137
  hot drinks, 135
  and rest, 130, 134
  sleeping pills, 130-133
  unlaxing muscles, 136-137
  warm baths, 135-136
Interests, and aging, 203-204
Intestinal disturbances, 62
Iodine, 56, 125, 142, 151-152, 168
Iridectomy, 184
Iron, in diet, 99
Isometric exercises, 87-88
Isotonic exercises, 87
Itching, 149

J

Japan, 48, 204
Jenner, William, 27

K

Kenny, Elizabeth ("Sister Kenny"), 25-
  28
Kickapoo Indian Salve, 139-140, 146, 148
Kidney secretion, 169
Kirkendall, Dr. Lester A., 200, 202
Knee flexing exercise, 82
Knee push exercise, 85

L

Lacrimal glands, 177
Lane, Dr., 151
Lanolin, 143
Laryngitis, 169-170
Laryngoscope, 27

Laughter, 198
Laxatives, 98-101, 151
Laymen, medical discoveries by, 27-28
Lecithin, 92
Leg lift exercise, 85
Leucocytes (white cells), 32
Life, prolongation of, 203-205
Life expectancy, 104, 195
Life Expectancy (table), 104
Light therapy (*See also* Sunbathing;
    Sunlamps; Ultraviolet radiation)
    advantages, 37
    biophysics of, 38
    effect on skin, 38-39
    and eyes, 37
    infrared, 42
Liver, 80, 132, 164
Liver oil, fish, 56
Living, zest for, 204
Longevity, 148-149
Lugol's solution, 125
Lupus vulgaris, 55
Lying down exercise, 81-87
Lymphoid tissues, 172-173
Lysozyme, 178

M

Malt soup extract, 101
"Man and Civilization; The Family's
    Search for Survival," 200
Manual massage *vs.* mechanical, 44
Marezine, 190
Margarines, 117
Marriage, and health, 199, 200-202
Massage:
    effleurage, 44-45
    friction, 46-47
    at home, 42-48
    manual *vs.* mechanical, 44
    massotherapy, 44-48
    for muscle cramps, 43-44
    in other countries, 48
    petrissage, 45-46
    and poor circulation, 45
    self-massage, 43
    tapotement, 47-48
    vibration, 47
Massotherapy, 44-48 *see also* Massage
Mastoiditis, 165, 193-194
Meals, scheduling of, 96-98 *see also*
    Diet
Meat:
    grading system, 117
    infested, 95-96
    saturated fat content, 117

Medical Center, University of Cali-
    fornia, 200
Medical discoveries, by laymen, 27-28
Melanin, 39
Meniere's Syndrome, 190
Menstrual periods, and sex, 201
Menthol, 143, 164
Metabolism, 65, 73-74
Middle-ear diseases, 165 *see also* Ears
Migraine, 190-191
Milk:
    allergy to, 92
    breast, 95
    and constipation, 99
    low-calorie products, 116-117
    pasteurization, 95
    from soya beans, 92
Milk of magnesia, 164
Milk products, low-calorie, 116-117
Milk sickness, 27-28
Mineral oil, 151
Minneapolis, Minn., Kenny method in,
    26
Moist cold compresses, 31-32
Motion sickness, 189-190
Mucous membranes, 64, 156
Mulford Colloid Laboratories, 144
Muscle cramps, massage for, 43-44
Mycin ointments, 183
Myotics, 184

N

Napoleon, 134
Narcotics, 130-133
Naso-lachrymal ducts, 178
Natural foods, 92
Natural laxatives, 98-101
Nausea, 124
Neoaristocort ophthalmic ointment, 183
Neomycin, 182, 183, 191
Neosynephrin, 157, 158-159
New York Society for Physical Medi-
    cine, 27
New York Times, 66
Newton, Isaac, 158, 191
Niacin, 190, 191
Niacinamide, 190
Nicotine, 132
Nicotinic Acid, 191 *see also* Niacin
Night blindness, 143
Nose:
    allergies, 158
    anatomy, 156-157
    blowing, 164-165
    colds *see* Colds

Nose (*cont.*)
  hayfever, 158
  nasal meati, 157
  nasal sprays, 157-158, 164
  nose drops, 158-159
  rhinitis medicamentosa, 158
  smoker's drip, 159
  and throat ailments, 170
  turbinates, 156, 157, 158
Nude bathing, 49-56
Nudity, social attitudes towards, 49-53
Nutritive oils, for skin, 55-56

O

Ocean bathing, 63-64, 66-67
Oil of sesame, 142
Oil of wintergreen, 60
Oils:
  fish, 56, 112
  olive, 56, 70, 149
  polyunsaturated, 112, 116, 117, 118
  vegetable, 56, 151
Oregon State University, 200
Organ meats, in diet, 112
Orient, fish consumption in, 112
Orient, massage in, 48
"Oriental milk," 92
Ormond Beach, Florida, 75
Osmosis, 33
Otitis Externa, 191
Otitis Media Catarrhalis Acuta, 193
Otomycosis, 145, 191
Overeating, 96, 97
Overweight *see* Reducing

P

Pain, hot packs for, 61
Para-aminobenzoic acid, 39, 70
Paraldehyde, 133
Parathyroid, 54
Parker's True Tonic, 155
Pasteurization, of milk, 95
Patent medicines, 139
Pectin, 99
Penicillin, 183
Peptic indigestion, 124-125
Peristalsis, 100
Peroxide, 153, 188
Persia, 27
Petrissage, 45-46 *see also* Massage
Photophobia, 40-41
Physical therapy, 25-29
Physiologic (natural) salt solution, 33
Pilocarpine, 184

Pimples, 55, 151-152
Pink eye, 179-180
Poison ivy, 143-144
Poliomyelitis, 25-28
Pollinosis, 158
Polyunsaturated fats, 112, 116, 117, 118
Pope, Alexander, 139
Pork, 95-96
Potassium iodide, 125
Potatoes, 94
Poultry, in diet, 112
Prescriptions *see* Rx's
Preventive medicine, 195
Privine, 157
Processed foods, 114-117
Protein in Common Foods (table), 108-109
Protein silver solution, 179, 180
Proteins, and ultraviolet rays, 38
Pruritus, 149
Psoriasis, 55

Q

Quinine, 163

R

Ragweed, 158
Raw food *vs.* cooked, 94-96
Reader's Digest, 27
Recreation, and exercise, 88-89
Reducing:
  Basic Daily Dietary, 91, 107-108
  bread and butter, 113
  butter substitutes, 116
  calorie allowance, daily, 105-107
  carbohydrates, 113
  crash diets, 103
  exercise, 85
  fish in diet, 111
  future diets, 118
  low-calorie processed foods, 114-117
  milk products, 116-117
  pound-a-week program, 107-114
  protein requirements, 108-109
  variety in menus, 110-112
  vitamins, 111 *see also* Vitamins
  weight, ideal, 104-105
Relaxation:
  daily program, 125-127
  eating habits, 120-121
  habits, fundamental, 120-121
  hot drinks, 121-123
  sleep, 136-137
Resistance exercises, 87-88

Respiratory infections, 62, 155-165 *see also* Colds; Nose; Throat ailments
Rest, 130, 134, 170
Restaurants, and diet, 97-98
Retirement, 202-203
Rhinitis medicamentosa, 158 *see also* Nose
Rhus toxicodendrum, 144
Riboflavin, 92 *see also* Vitamins
Right angle exercise, 87
Rockefeller, John D., Sr., 75
Romans, eating habits, 96
Roosevelt, Franklin D., 76
Roosevelt, Theodore, 179
Roughage, in diet, 99
Rx's (prescriptions):
    air bathing, 72-73
    Aveeno Oilated baths, 150
    baldness, 147-148
    belly breathing, 79
    black eyes, 178-179
    boils, 152
    cold cream, 141
    cold water therapy, 58-59
    colds, 163-164
    constipation, 101
    cough syrup, 168
    earache, 192
    ear wax, 188-189
    halitosis, 171
    hot drinks for relaxation, 121
    hot foot baths, 61-62
    hot hypertonic salt solution, 34
    hot water therapy, 60
    indigestion, 123
    insecticides, removal of, 93
    laxative, 101
    migraine, 190-191
    mosit cold compresses, 32
    muscle cramps, 43-44
    nausea, 124
    peptic indigestion, 124
    pink eye, 179
    salt bath, 62-63
    Silvers' Swab Solution, 168
    sinus headaches, 157
    smoker's drip, 159
    tired eyes, 182-183
    trench mouth, 171

S

Sabin vaccine, 26
Safety rules, ocean bathing, 66-67
Salicylic acid, 142 *see also* Aspirin
Salivary glands, 156

Salk vaccine, 26
Salt solutions, hypertonic, 33-34
Salt solutions, physiologic, 33
Salt water bathing, at home, 62-63
Scandinavia, 48
Scissors exercise, 86
Sea air, 63
Seafood, 125
Seasickness, 124
Seborrhoea, 147
Sebum, 143, 188
Self-massage, 43
Senility, premature, 204
Sense of balance, 189-190
Sense of humor, 198
Sesame oil, 149
Sex, in marriage, 200-202
Sex education, in schools, 200
Shellfish, Composition of (table), 111
Shortness of breath, after exercising, 84
Shoulder curling exercise, 82
Showers, exercise after, 81
Sight *see* Eyes
Silvers, Myra, 27
Silvers' Swab Solution, 168, 172
Sinuses, 34, 156, 157-158, 165
Sit-up exercise, 84
Skimmed milk, 116
Skin:
    acne, 149
    aging, 148-150
    air conditioning, 150
    "athletes foot" of, 144-145
    Aveeno, 149-150
    baldness, 146-148
    boils, 151-152
    burns, 145-146
    cold cream, 141-142, 149
    colloidal emollient baths, 149-150
    constipation, 150-151
    cosmetics, 139-142
    dermatophytosis, 144-145
    dermis, 150
    egg white, 153
    epidermis, 150
    fungoid growths, 144-145
    hats, effect on scalp, 147
    hives, 144
    ichthyosis, 142
    injuries, 153-154
    itching, 149
    laxatives, 151
    light therapy, 38-39, 50, 54-55
    mineral oil, 151
    moisture, 150
    nude bathing, 49-56

Skin (*cont.*)
nutrition, 55-56
oil balance, 143
oils for, 149
otomycosis, 145, 191
pimples, 151-152
poison ivy, 143-144
pruritus, 149
psychological factors, 143
scaly skin, 142-143
seborrhoea, 147
sebum, 143
soap, 149
Sleep, 129-137 *see also* Insomnia
Sleep habit pattern, 120
Sleeping pills, 130-133
Smoker's drip, 159
Smoking, 132, 133, 159, 164
Snakeroot, 28
Snow blindness, 40
Soaps, and skin, 149
Sodium bicarbonate, 164, 189
Sodium perborate, 171, 172
Sore throats *see* Throat ailments
Soya beans, 92
Spa bathing, at home, 60-61
"Speaker's sore throat," 169
Sprains, 46
Sprays, nasal, 157-158, 164
Stammerers and stutterers, 80
Stare, Dr. Frederick, 115
Steroids, 144
Stomach, excess acid in, 123
Stratum corneum, of skin, 39
Stretch-over exercise, 83
Styes, 183
Sulpha drugs, 192
Sulphathiazole gum, 171
Sunbathing, 39-41, 69-76, 142 *see also* Light therapy
Sunburn, 39-41
Sunburn, of the eyes, 40-41
Sunlamp therapy, 50
Sunlamps, selection and use, 54-55
Suntan lotions, 39, 70
Sweating, 145, 163, 169
Swimming, and ear infections, 192-194
Swimming, as exercise, 80-81

T

Tachypnea, 84
Talcum, borated, 145
Tanning, of skin, 39, 55, 69-70 *see also* Light therapy; Sunbathing; Sunlamps; Ultraviolet radiation

Tapotement, 47-48 *see also* Massage
Tarsal glands, 178
Tea, 121, 135
Tears, 177-178 *see also* Eyes
Temperature, in hydrotherapy, 57-58
Temperature-Humidity Index, 65-66
Tetanus, 153, 154
Thiamin, 92 *see also* Vitamins
Throat ailments, 167-175
cough medicines, 167-169
gargling, 168-169, 170, 171
hot salt solutions, 170
laryngitis, 169-170
nose, 170
rest, 170
"speaker's sore throat," 169
steam inhalations, 170
swabs, 168
tonsils, 172-175
Tissue inflammation, 144
Tobacco *see* Smoking
Tonsils, 172-175
Tranquilizers, 136
Trench mouth, 170-171
Triamcinolone, 144, 182, 191
Trichinosis, 95-96
Turbinates, of nose, 156, 157, 158
Twain, Mark, 59

U

Ulcers, 123
Ultraviolet radiation, 38, 55, 72-73, 142, 174 *see also* Light therapy; Sunbathing; Sunlamps
Undecylenic acid, 145

V

Vacations, 198-199
Vaccination, 27
Vaporizers, 170
Varicose veins, 80
Variety meats, in diet, 112
Vascular diseases, 92, 112, 164, 197
Veal, in diet, 112
Vegetable oils, 56, 151
Vesiculation, 39
Vibratory massage, 47 *see also* Massage
Viosterol *see* Vitamin D
Viruses, of common cold, 160
Vitamins:
A, 56, 92, 143, 151
B_1, 92, 94

Vitamins *(cont.)*
  B₂, 92
  B Complex, 92, 111
  brewer's yeast, 92
  D, 38, 54, 55, 56, 69, 70, 72, 73, 92,
      142, 151
  in diet, 92
  E, 56, 94, 151
  fat soluble, 56, 151
  K, 56, 151
  and metabolism, 74
  Niacin, 190, 191
  P, 94
  and reducing, 111
  requirements, daily, 91

W

Warm baths, for insomnia, 135-136
Warner, Charles Dudley, 75

Water therapy *(See also* Baths)
  benefits of, 57-58
  cold water, 58-59
  hot water, 59-61
  ocean bathing, 63-64
  salt water, at home, 62-63
  temperature, 57-58
Wax, in ears, 188-189
Weather, best use of, 75-76
Weight *see* Reducing
Wheat germ, 92
White Beaver's Cough Cream, 155
White cells (leucocytes), 32
Wigs, 146-147, 148
Wright, Frank Lloyd, 148
Wives and husbands, 199-202

Z

Zirconium oxide, 143